Praise for *The Inside Story*

"Rejoice! Susan Sands has crafted an exquisitely written, indispensable antidote to the inexorable fear and revulsion attendant to the aging process, especially with respect to body image. Eschewing the typical self-help promise of triumph over aging, Sands deftly provides an integrated guide to navigating and enriching the aging process, utilizing a groundbreaking weaving of neuroscience and psychology that upends our fraught expectations about living in an aging body. With depth and grace, she turns our thinking about women aging on its head, challenging us to think about aging not as a problem or disorder but as a fresh and novel way to live in a stable older body. Sands invigorates our minds with the hope of finding solace and fertile ground through remaking and reexperiencing our relationship to our bodies so that we can live in and from them, in their 'glory' or not, as is."

Jean Petrucelli, PhD, CEDS
editor of *Body-States* and director of EDCAS at The
William Alanson White Institute

"We might wish to scorn our aging, but Susan Sands invites us to understand and—yes!—even relish our embodiments' many surprises and gifts. This is a work of love to women."

Susie Orbach
author of *Fat is a Feminist Issue* and *Bodies*

"A delicious brew of new knowledge and fresh ideas, seasoned with a feminism that spans a long, rich life. What a treat!"

Valory Mitchell, PhD
coauthor of the 50-year study *Women on the River of Life*

"Now more than ever, we want to inhabit our bodies comfortably, honor our cycles, and consciously evolve. As we grow older, Susan's book makes the neurological and psychological case for tending to the most vital relationship of all—with ourselves."

Elena Brower
author of *Being You*

"Every woman over 50 must read this book; it will transform their lives. Dr. Sands's core message is that women do not just have a body, they are a body, and being able to know and feel their bodies from the inside is the gateway to contentment and full acceptance of their aging. Supported by the latest neuroscience research and full of gripping first-person accounts of women struggling to come to terms with growing older, The Inside Story offers many practical methods—from mindfulness to touch, movement and yoga—for women to know themselves not for what others say they are, but for who they truly are, inside and out."

Lewis Richmond
author of *Aging as a Spiritual Practice*

The
Inside Story

The
Inside Story

The Surprising
Pleasures of Living
in an Aging Body

Susan Sands, PhD

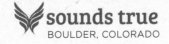

BOULDER, COLORADO

Sounds True
Boulder, CO 80306

Published 2022

Cover design by Jennifer Miles
Book design by Meredith March

The wood used to produce this book is from
Forest Stewardship Council (FSC) certified forests,
recycled materials, or controlled wood.

Printed in Canada

BK06232

Library of Congress Cataloging-in-Publication Data

Names: Sands, Susan (Psychologist), author.
Title: The inside story : the surprising pleasures of living in an aging body
   / by Susan Sands, PhD.
Description: Boulder, CO : Sounds True, 2022. | Includes bibliographical
   references and index.
Identifiers: LCCN 2021036480 (print) | LCCN 2021036481 (ebook) | ISBN
   9781683648093 (hardback) | ISBN 9781683648109 (ebook)
Subjects: LCSH: Aging--Psychological aspects. | Aging–Physiological
   aspects. | Older women–Psychology. | Body image. | Self-esteem in old age.
Classification: LCC BF724.8 .S26 2022 (print) | LCC BF724.8 (ebook) | DDC
   155.67–dc23
LC record available at https://lccn.loc.gov/2021036480
LC ebook record available at https://lccn.loc.gov/2021036481

10 9 8 7 6 5 4 3 2 1

Contents

Introduction

I woke this morning to balmy air, a clear sky, and a burning desire to head out with the dog to the eucalyptus-shaded trail near my home in the Berkeley hills. As I always do these days, I first stretch the kinks out of my knees, ankles, and back. Then I carefully make my way down the dusty, rutted hill at the start of the trail, placing each foot firmly. The light is filtering through the cathedral of trees in a particularly glorious way this morning, and as I look up and lock into that beauty, my foot hits a small rock and I lurch. "Watch your footing!" I hiss to myself under my breath. This sense of cautiousness is with me more these days. I'm in pretty good shape, but at seventy-four I know I have to watch it. I'm not the invincible forty-five-year-old I used to be. I can feel age creeping slowly through my body—nothing major, but a bit slower on the uptake, a tad weaker, an ankle that acts up if I don't keep it strong, a bit less sure of my balance.

The facts are incontrovertible. I was born and will age and die like every other human being and every other living thing on the planet. No exceptions. I have no choice about this. How I age, however, is where I have some choice, although there will also be plenty of surprises and no say whatsoever about the outcome. As I gaze up at the eucalyptus trees, which, like me, are aging by living, I know that my sanest choice is not to protest or deny the inevitable but to get to know and make friends with my aging body. I need to develop a new, healthier relationship with my older body; or, more accurately, I need to develop a relationship with my *new* body, my new aging body.

When not on the hiking trail, I have, for the past thirty-five years, been thinking deeply about women's bodies. As a clinical psychologist,

I've been teaching, training, publishing articles, and doing psychotherapy centered on body-based difficulties, like eating disorders, as well as aging. The "body sense" is what I'm most interested in—the body we feel and experience *from within*. I'm particularly interested in promoting the integration of mind and body, which allows us to have the invigorating sense of actually *living* in the body, what we call "embodiment." Western civilization has been, until very recently, so strangely focused on the mind to the exclusion of the body, when, in truth, the body is the foundation of all of our experience from birth until death.

It is now scientifically established that our minds are rooted in our bodies. Our minds are formed through sensing and feeling our moving bodies as they interact with the environment, especially the important people around us. Our emotional awareness, our sense of well-being, our very sense of "self" is created from our inner body sensations! In other words, the future of "you" depends on how well you attend to and process all the crucial information streaming from within your body.

Yet, hardly any scientists or scholars are asking how our body experience affects how we *age*—even though the body is the visible evidence, bellwether, and "messenger" of aging! The aging female body, as women *experience* it—whether comfortably or uncomfortably, positively or negatively—is still routinely ignored, rendering it irrelevant or unthinkable. I passionately believe that our inner body experience is of utmost importance as we age, and I will urge you to develop your body awareness as the best way to get to know, accept, and enjoy your older body.

In this book, we will look at aging through a focus on the body, based on cutting-edge neuroscience and psychology, which will transform your view of your aging body and your later years. How do we know we have a body? How does the body sense develop? How do we create our emotions out of body sensations? How do we develop body awareness? How does our body sense change as we age? What happens to our sense of self when we don't feel comfortable in our body, especially as we age?

One of my interviewees told me, with a little smile, "I'm so much more comfortable in my body at sixty-eight than I was in my twenties or thirties, even though I look older." She was describing the pleasurable experience of being embodied, at home in her body, sensing her body from within.

What allows my interviewee to override the dictates of our youth-obsessed, image-saturated culture? What makes it possible for this particular woman to feel comfortable in her body, while so many of us feel fear, sadness, anger, or shame in this ageist, Botoxing, tummy-tucking society? Why are so many of us so *disconnected* from our bodies—so focused on how our bodies look rather than how they feel? Why do we continue to focus on our appearance rather than our experience *even as we age*, when we become more physically vulnerable and must take excellent care of our somatic selves? These are essential, unaddressed questions, which I'll explore in this book, as we begin to reflect on our sense of ourselves from the inside out.

This book is not about trying to look fifty when you're seventy or thirty when you're fifty or training to run marathons at eighty—unless you're the outlier who really wants to and can. It's not a book about trying to stop the clock. It is, instead, a book about forging a healthier relationship with your *actual* maturing body—a relationship not of fear, hatred, or shame but of respect, appreciation, tenderness, and, yes, even love. I want to help you create an older yet still positive and vital sense of your body that you can live with for the rest of your life.

I believe we older women are actually *primed* to experience our bodies more deeply and pleasurably. Our bodies are quieter and slower. There is less dramatic action inside the theater of our bodies without the cyclical changes of our younger years. There are also certain brain changes that come with aging that allow our bodies to become less reactive, particularly to negative stimuli, and give rise to a greater sense of well-being. Aging can thus open up a transformational and pleasurable new capacity for body awareness, allowing many women to become truly embodied only in older age.

But . . . are you perhaps thinking at this point that this is a perfect book for your mother or grandmother and doesn't really apply to you? Think again if you're forty-five or over. As a perimenopausal woman, you're entering the second half of your life, a time when you should assess where you are and where you're going. And if you're beyond or well beyond menopause, there's no time like the present to rethink your relationship with your body. How comfortable you are *with* and *in* your aging body has a huge impact on how you feel about yourself as you grow older.

I am at the leading edge of the Baby Boomer generation, which includes almost forty million American women aged fifty-seven to seventy-five. Driven by the aging of the Boomers, the number of people over sixty-five has grown by over a *third* since 2010 and will make up 20 percent of the nation's population by 2030, compared with 13 percent in 2010. The fastest-growing age group is eighty-five years and older. We older folks make up a powerful new demographic, with women increasingly outnumbering men.[1]

We're living longer and longer, and we need help negotiating the profoundly altered sense of the body that comes with aging. We feel both like the same person we've always been and yet remarkably different. Sometimes it's almost eerie—that woman in the mirror doesn't match the one we see in our mind's eye. We have to *learn* how to age—from confronting our mortality to the nitty-gritty of learning to live in a changing body. Our society offers few "instructions" for these years, unlike in earlier stages when our "tasks" (like school, marriage, child-rearing, and career) are laid out for us.[2] What are the tasks of older age? What do we need to learn to live wisely? How can we make peace with—even *friends* with—our older bodies? While I don't want to downplay the real and sometimes difficult physical and mental disabilities that can accompany aging, I do want to show that we have a lot of choice about how to guide our precious bodies through the unpredictable terrain of our later years, changes you might start seeing as early as age forty-five.

To do this, we need to have a sense that we are standing shoulder to shoulder with other women going through the same process, who will "tell it like it is." Here is the Polish poet Wislawa Szymborska talking about how her poetry was changed by the upheaval of World War II. She could just as easily be describing the way we are changed by aging: "It was not possible to use the same language as before. We all felt the need to use a very simple, very brash language. We wanted poetry without artifice."[3]

I include throughout the book the "simple, brash" language of the thirty women I have interviewed, as well as my patients and friends, all of whom range in age from forty-eight to ninety-one years and in ethnic, socioeconomic, and health status. There are many different paths through the tangled aging terrain, and I will let these women speak for themselves about how they've experienced their bodies from childhood to the present and how they've thrown off the negative, constricting body messages from earlier years, like a coat that no longer fits, and found renewed pride and pleasure in their bodies as they age. I acknowledge the real and sometimes difficult physical and mental disabilities that can accompany aging and have interviewed women with both with lifelong and recent disabilities. My fervent hope is that my book will help women of diverse abilities, circumstances, outlooks, and gender identities create an accepting yet still vibrant sense of their older bodies.

Because it's so easy to think of our aging bodies as a jumble of aches and pains and sags and losses, I will endeavor to help us understand and appreciate all the extraordinary things the body does for us beyond those physical functions that can become compromised as we age. When we appreciate the breadth and majesty of our body's offerings, we counteract our society's obsessive preoccupation with physical appearance.

One of the most amazing bodily processes is what's called "interoception," the science of how we sense ourselves from within. Internal sensory signals streaming from all over the body get integrated in different parts of our brains until they are ultimately mapped in a special part of our cortex called the "insula," which gives us a sense of the condition of our entire body, which, in turn, allows us to feel emotion and maintain our sense of "self."[4] The exciting new science of interoception has the power to transform our vision of what we are and who we can be as we get older. Strong "interoceptive awareness" also helps us take good care of our bodies as we age. Our evolving understanding of the body's central role in "neuroplasticity"—the ability of the brain to change and grow—also has wide repercussions for older age.

In our current blatantly ageist, media-saturated culture, the ideal twenty-first-century Western woman is perennially stuck—like Dorian Gray—in an eighteen- to twenty-three-year-old body. Even if you're a vibrant forty-eight, you're seen by many as "an older woman." What is new and particularly insidious is that the body is now viewed as a crucial personal "project"[5] to be honed, altered, and transformed through exercise, dieting, cosmetic surgery, injections, implants, peels, and, more recently, Photoshop. The number of cosmetic surgeries in the United States more than doubled between 2000 and 2015, and the biggest increase is in those under thirty who are opting for "early maintenance" to avoid larger procedures later on.[6] Why is our society so fixated on the young female body? Why do we seem to need to control and alter women's bodies? It's a difficult time in history to feel comfortable in a body of *any* age, much less an older body. My aim is to disrupt this sorry scenario and help us take our bodies back.

How can we manage the multiple losses of aging without disappointment, anger, disgust, and shame? I will urge you to stop focusing on the "outside body," which others *see*—the one you may think is too fat, too wrinkled, or too saggy—and move your attention to what I call the "inside body," which you sense and feel. When you pay more attention to your body sensations—such as the ache in your lower back, which signals it's time to rest—you actually build more neural connections in those parts of your brain that monitor internal sensations and thus become more adept at living in and nurturing your body. The burgeoning new body science helps counter our culture's terrible fear of aging, instead transforming our vision of who we can be as we age.

Our fear and hatred of aging is part of our much broader cultural problem—what I call the "triumphing over the body" narrative, which is related to the "triumphing over nature," "triumphing over aging," and, ultimately, "triumphing over death" narratives. I think of actor Carrie Fisher, at age fifty-five, dancing with great effort up a ladder in heels in her one-woman show, "Wishful Drinking." Women's narratives, we shall see, usually have to do with conquering the *body*. And we keep trying to find "solutions" to the "problem" of aging, as if it were a disorder. I particularly love this passage from Ram Dass: "It is as if we are urged to fight over and over again a losing battle against time, pitting ourselves against natural law. How ghastly this is, and how inhumane, toward both ourselves and the cycle of life. It reminds me of someone rushing around the fields in the autumn painting the marvelous gold and red leaves with green paint."[7]

Triumphing over the body is not a good narrative for us as we age. It's not a good idea to ignore or subjugate our bodies at the very time that they are becoming more vulnerable and need special attention and care.

We need, instead, to develop a more respectful and loving relationship with our bodies, and I offer strategies to help you inhabit your older body with more ease and equanimity.

We will also delve into the nitty-gritty of how to live well in an aging body. I lay out the scientific findings on the benefits and the "how to" of increasing our body awareness through Eastern body practices like meditation and yoga and breath work. The benefits are stunning, including better emotional regulation, sharper concentration, greater empathy, firmer emotional "boundaries," and more overall happiness. There is a direct physiological link, research shows, between being aware of your body and being able to regulate your body functions and restore your physical and emotional health. I will show you how body awareness made me more able to "fix" parts of my body that weren't functioning properly. Finally, I will encourage you to really *enjoy* your body and offer suggestions about how to embrace the distinctive beauty of every age and discover and embody your unique attractiveness.

It was striking to me that all of the women I interviewed for this book told me, without being asked, that their lives had gotten *better* in many ways with age. Burgeoning research shows that aging spurs new psychological development in later life, including greater happiness, emotional regulation, and optimism, with age eighty-two being the year of greatest happiness![8] It is also my strong belief that the shedding of the veils that accompanies a true encounter with our mortality allows us to truly accept the reality of our lives—including the reality of our aging bodies—in a way not before possible.[9] Seeing ourselves as part of the larger cycle of life allows us to feel more profoundly connected to other human beings and the natural world. These new capacities do not make up for, but do soften and buffer, the many losses of the aging process. If we're clear-eyed about our mortality, confront our fears, and settle comfortably into our bodies, we can move from a focus on who we *were* to who we're *becoming*.

Imagine this. What if we became part of a movement to transform our society's dismal view of aging? Our older generations have successfully advocated for the rights of women and people of every color, sexual and gender orientation, and disability. But the universal human process of *aging* remains a human rights frontier! What if we could help usher in a different view of our aging bodies, one more like that in Asia, where elders are not expected to have youthful bodies and are treated with admiration and celebration?

This book will help get us there. When you grasp that your bodily, "lived" experience is the very foundation of your self-awareness, emotional life, and well-being, you'll appreciate it more and attend to it more carefully. When you assimilate the burgeoning science on the benefits of meditation, yoga, and breath work, you'll become more motivated to pursue these transformative body practices. As you get more comfortable with and in your maturing body, you'll be better able to face the perfectly normal process of aging and death. When you learn about the multiple, surprising *benefits* of growing older, you can challenge our society's profound ageism (including your own) and see your last stage of life as an essential and illuminating one. I invite you to join me in creating a more positive, even proud, sense of your aging body, as you delve into *the inside story* of your life.

Chapter 1

Living in the Body

The studio in North Berkeley was small, steamy, and dimly lit, yet the air was alive with energy. The women around me, in their fifties, sixties, and seventies, were stretching and laughing, their powerful, bare arms and shoulders glowing in the soft light. Their voices resonated deep in their chests; they stood erect, with straight spines and heads held high. They radiated health and joy. They were magnificent! What was going on here? I felt as if I had landed on another planet inhabited by superwomen.

Earlier in the week, I had signed up for a class for older women on "strengthening the pelvic floor," and, somehow, I had ended up in a class filled with master yoga teachers! As I unrolled my mat and sat down, I found myself stealing glances at a powerfully built woman in a lime-green leotard who seemed to move with no effort at all. Years later, I can still see her and feel the energy of that room. By slowly and radically training her body over time, she had actually changed her body, as well as her presence, her energy, and her very being.

This experience, from more than a decade ago, made a huge impression on me. I felt so awed, yet so different and so removed from these powerful women. Yes, as a kid I'd been active in sports in school, and as an adult I've done running, tennis, skiing, swimming, workouts, yoga, and lots of hiking. But I had never really taken my body as seriously as my mind—except for its appearance, of course. I hadn't conceived of my body as something to be deeply listened to, taken care of, and carefully developed. I didn't yet know that feeling rooted in my body in an ongoing way was crucial to my sense of well-being. I felt such admiration for those yoga teachers, who had so deliberately and devotedly dedicated themselves to their bodies.

I've also had my lifelong disappointments with my body, of course—too "boyish," not curvy enough, hands and feet too wide, hair too frizzy, and so forth—and it certainly didn't help that my mother never seemed comfortable with her own sexuality. Doubtless you, like most women, have your own issues with your body. Was your mom always putting you on the scale? Or maybe when you'd walk into the living room all dressed up, your dad wouldn't even notice you? Did your brother and his friends call you "meatball"? Have you spent your life dreading seeing your reflection in shop windows? Or maybe you had terrible period cramps or a particularly difficult childbirth, from which your body never seemed to recover. Or you experienced sexual abuse or physical abuse or traumatic injuries or surgeries, so now your body feels like a dangerous place to inhabit. Perhaps when your teenage daughter became anorexic, you could recognize in her something of your own hatred of your body. Or maybe you saw your mother injure her back and then, following doctor's orders, put on a back brace and slowly descend into disability, which she called "getting old."

No wonder you came to see your body as something to be rejected or ignored. No wonder you developed a fundamental *mind-body disconnect*. So then, perhaps, you focused more exclusively on academic or workplace achievement or social status, and you've never thought very much about your physical body. It just operates silently in the background. And when the yoga teacher says, "activate your abs," you have no idea what she's talking about or how to do it. Or perhaps you did finally begin to pay attention to your body when you sprained your knee and had to go to physical therapy and learned more about how your body is put together (like how a hip misalignment caused your knee injury), and you wished that you had understood all that earlier. The fact is that when most of us were growing up, our physical bodies *as we experienced them* (as opposed to our appearance) were not really focused on or valued. If you're a Boomer or older, there were few intramural sports for girls, and no one really "went to the gym" outside of school, nor did we do Eastern bodily practices like yoga or meditation or tai chi, except maybe as a lark, some "new thing." And, of course, no matter what age you are, it's been difficult for most any female, living under the "male gaze" in our hyper-sexualized and misogynistic culture, to feel truly comfortable in her body. I remember "training" myself as a teenager to make my movements more "mincing" and less confident and to lean back and thrust my hips forward to make myself shorter.

We've learned to dismiss or hate or fear our bodies for many different and individual reasons, of course, but a crucial but unrecognized factor is that we've never really gotten to *know* our bodies, to sense and feel our bodies from the inside out. In our society, connection to our bodies (except sex) or to the natural world is downplayed and undervalued unless you're a serious athlete. "Success" has meant developing your thinking self at the expense of your body self—your "conceptual self-awareness" rather than your "somatic self-awareness." As babies, of course, we were all-body, but then "maturing" meant gradually losing that body awareness. We never learned how to read and interpret sensations arising from within our bodies and to use this information to make decisions about what we need and want. The result is that too many of us are left with a mind-body disconnect that keeps us from knowing ourselves deeply. This is particularly dangerous for us as we age, when we become more physically vulnerable and need to take excellent care of ourselves.

Now, as you move through the second half of your life, you have another wide-open opportunity to reconnect mind and body and to create a healthier relationship with your body. Just because you've treated your body in a certain way until now doesn't mean you have to continue to do that as an older adult. You can keep on reshaping how you feel about and *in* your body until the very end. You may prefer to work primarily in a physical way with your body, like the yoga teachers, or you may find yourself working more psychologically with your attitudes about your body, like my interviewee Elizabeth.

Elizabeth, a fast-talking seventy-four-year-old with piercing blue eyes, told me about her own fascinating evolution as we sat together at my kitchen table munching rye crisp and hummus, while rain pattered on the skylight:

> When I started growing around eleven or twelve, I kept getting taller and taller, and my mother just couldn't stand it. She was so worried about me. She would keep track of my height by marking it in pencil on the closet door. She particularly didn't like my long legs. She had this thing about my extremely long thighs. By the time I was thirteen, I was taller than she was and somehow that was the last straw. One time, she stood on the stairs, put her hands on my shoulders, pushed down hard and actually said, "Stop growing or no one will marry you!" (When I asked Elizabeth if her mother was joking, she said no, her mother was perfectly serious.) I just kept growing, and I kept losing hope. I really hated my body as a teenager. I just studied. I didn't dare to even think that any boys could like me in high school and even in college. I started going out some but always wearing flats. It wasn't until my late twenties that I felt attractive at all.

Elizabeth has since "grown into" her height of 5'10" and, at seventy-four, is a strikingly vivacious and attractive woman. She is married to a loving tall man who adores her. After many years of psychotherapy and body therapy, she knows herself well. I was particularly struck by one of the last things Elizabeth said in our interview, as the rain pounded on the darkening skylight. We were talking about what she wants for herself now, and she said, "I want to be a wilder older woman and have more dramatic clothes and a streak in my hair. I think my goal is to be a little bit larger-than-life older woman!" It appears that Elizabeth has taken her mother's fears, so hurtful originally, and upended them. She now wants to transform her tallness into another very appealing kind of largeness.

Of course, if we engage with our bodies in *both* ways—physically, like the yoga teachers, and emotionally, like Elizabeth—we have the best chance of chugging happily into the later chapters of our lives. I strongly believe—and my experience shows me—that with some knowledge and guidance you can become more adept at knowing viscerally what's happening in your body and what it needs and desires. You can *rediscover* that ability to sense yourself you had as a baby and then lost. Then you'll be able to more easily regulate your body functions and restore your physical and emotional health. If you learn to take care of yourself with respect and tenderness, you can feel more connected to and comfortable in your body and in yourself now than you ever have before. In fact, as we shall see, some of us can make peace with our bodies *only* in older age.

Am I suggesting that we can learn to find our older bodies as pleasing as our younger ones? No, that's asking way too much. What I am saying is that we can create a better, more loving *relationship* with our bodies. We can finally become friends rather than adversaries. For it is still the case that the majority of us are uncomfortable with our aging bodies. One recent study of two thousand women over age fifty (average age fifty-nine) found that only 12 percent felt satisfied with their body size,[1] and a report from the American Society of Plastic Surgeons reveals that cosmetic procedures for Americans over age fifty-five rose 28 percent since 2010.[2] And while research also shows that many women worry less about size and appearance as they move further into old age,[3] it is a sad fact that many women continue to have negative, even hateful, feelings toward their bodies. Ageism, not age, is the cause of these negative feelings. Our peace of mind in our later years is determined to no small degree by how well we get along with our corporeal selves. Wouldn't it be wonderful if we could all feel more like my seventy-five-year-old interviewee Judy, who said, with tears in her eyes, "I feel so incredibly grateful to my body, my sweet body . . . still faithful after all these years."

In this and the following chapters, I will lay out a new and surprising way of looking at the body and the development of the body that I believe opens up a fresh approach to the challenges of growing older. This basic body knowledge—all based on the latest science—can help us understand and appreciate what our bodies do for us and what our bodies need.

The Body Sense

The body is suddenly big news, after many years of being a bit player in the study of human development. Scholars and scientists from many different disciplines, including psychology, neuroscience, psychoanalysis, and philosophy, have started to ask similar questions about the body. What is the body? How do we know we have a body? How does it develop? What is the relationship of body and mind? How do we become embodied—that is, how do we come to feel at home in our body? What happens to our sense of self when we don't feel comfortable in our body? I ask an additional crucial question: How does our comfort or discomfort with our body affect how we age?

Our sense of having a body is not "natural" or inherent.[4] Babies are not born with a sense of "my body." We only gradually come to experience ourselves as having bodies, and we only gradually develop a sense of having an inside and an outside. I call this experience of bodily self-awareness the *body sense* (or, sometimes, the *body self* or *embodied self*). We have a strong and positive body sense if we have the ability to pay attention to our sensations, emotions, movements, and position in space, in the present moment. A strong body sense does not just "happen": it must be actively attended to, cultivated, and renewed.

Why do I focus here on "body sense" rather than on the more commonly discussed term "body image"? I do so because body image refers mainly to our imagined body, how we picture ourselves in our minds, whereas I want to focus on the feel, the experience, the awareness we have (or don't have) of our actual bodies. It takes a while—for some people a very long time, *if ever*—to develop a sense of really "residing" in our bodies, what I'm calling being "embodied."[5]

A good example is my patient Laurie, who is small and pixie-like but whose feet seem firmly planted on the ground and whose movements are confident. She can tell you how her body is feeling and how she is doing emotionally. When something's not feeling good, she often knows what's wrong and how to fix it. If her right hip is hurting, she knows exactly how to stretch it out; if she's feeling frantic about her drug-dependent daughter, she knows exactly the right friend to call to talk her down off the ledge. And it's not that her body or her health is perfect. Far from it. Laurie is in the middle stages of Parkinson's disease, and, despite this, she tries to take care of and love her body as much as she can. She exercises every day, as her doctors prescribed, and she eats nutritious food and sleeps nine hours every night. On the other hand, we saw in my interview with Elizabeth that a healthy body does not automatically produce a strong *sense* or a positive experience of the body. Although Elizabeth's body was from the beginning strong and beautiful, her mother's intense anxiety about her height led her to feel ungainly and unappealing, and she hated her body until she was well into her twenties. Only now, in her seventies, is Elizabeth really enjoying and feeling comfortable with her physical stature.

It is clear that how we feel about our bodies is not merely a reflection of how beautiful or strong or healthy or competent our bodies are. Rather, how we feel about our bodies depends to a large degree on how we feel *in* our bodies, which largely depends on how others have responded to our bodies throughout our life. We all know people who are "objectively" beautiful in appearance but who seem uncomfortable or self-conscious, and other people whose facial features or shape do not conform to our standards of perfection but who project a sense of ease and confidence that makes them attractive.

The significance of this integration of body and self, or "embodiment," for our well-being cannot be overemphasized. When we are embodied, easily feeling and sensing our body, we have the invigorating sense of actually *living* in our body, feeling connected to and "at home" in our body. We are in present time. All here. When we are firmly planted in our body, rather than in our thinking mind, we feel more grounded, clear, steady, and strong, with a greater sense of our own authority. We like and respect ourselves more and compare ourselves less to others. We are more psychologically healthy. Body and mind are experienced not as separate entities but as inseparable, a single unit. We're aware of our bodily feelings and sensations, internal and external, and we can use this knowledge to recognize our own needs and desires and to act on them.

It's also true, mounting research shows, that people who can pick up on and respond to signals from their bodies are considerably less likely to develop many debilitating physical and mental health conditions.[6] Why? Because they are able to become aware of minor physical problems earlier and treat those problems before they progress into chronic, serious conditions—for example, by tending to high blood sugar levels before they trigger diabetes.

Recent research also reveals that our body sense must be "constructed" slowly over time through countless interactions with our mothers and other caregivers and with our culture—a process I will discuss in depth in chapter 3. Indeed, our actual physical body, as well as our body sense, is also profoundly influenced or "shaped" by interactions and experiences with other people. Our posture, the comfort of our gut, the clarity of our skin, the tightness of our muscles—all are constantly being affected and shaped by what's happening to us and how we interpret these events. As infants, are we tenderly held, snuggled, soothed, played with, and delighted in . . . or not? How comfortable do our mothers feel in their own bodies, and how does their comfort or discomfort affect us? As we get older and go about our lives, do we feel accepted, respected, and cherished . . . or not? Are we sedentary, or engaged in lots of movement? Do we feel calm, or agitated? Bored, or stimulated? Overburdened, or carefree? All is reflected in the body. Imagine the bent shoulders and drooping eyelids of someone who feels lonely or overburdened, and the sparkling eyes and uplifted head of someone who feels connected to others and able to manage life's burdens. And how much are we influenced by our larger culture, with its disturbing focus on the young, thin, beautiful, and extreme, or its love affair with technology, where mental agility is glorified to the neglect of the body?

Shortly, we will delve more deeply into this fascinating process of how our body selves are created and shaped through relationships and the surrounding culture. But first, let's take a step back and consider how odd it is that the body—without which we are literally nothing, no*body*—has been given such a minor role in human development for so long.

The Body in the Shadows

The idea that from infancy on, our body and our body sense is shaped by human interactions and experiences is still novel for most people. While we have no trouble grasping that it takes a long time and a lot of outside input—twelve to twenty or more years of school!—for our brains and our personalities to develop, we somehow believe that our body develops according to an innate, preprogrammed process, which, barring defect, injury, or illness, will unfold automatically until we are adults. We all have a general genetic blueprint, of course. But the specifics of how our body develops depend significantly on many outside factors, such as how we interact with our caregivers and others and how we are influenced by our larger culture.

These groundbreaking new perspectives on the body unsettle a long history in which the body has played a minor role in human psychological development, at least in Western civilization. There are many complicated reasons for this history; I will mention three. The first is the Puritanism of our Judeo-Christian religious traditions. The "carnal" body has been seen as sinful—worthy even of flagellation or other mortification—and therefore not to be gratified. The second is our European philosophical tradition, epitomized by René Descartes, which holds that the essence of our being is located in our mind, not our body, and that mind and body are separate. This belief disregards the way the mind is "embedded" in the body, as well as in relationships, and in the natural world.[7] It pays no attention, for instance, to the fact that all of our emotions are experienced and generated in our body, before being "thought about" in the cortex of the brain.

Likewise, even in the fields specifically devoted to the subject of aging, the physical body is separated from its environment[8]: the body resides in geriatrics, a medical specialty focused on the care and treatment of older people, while the psychological and social dimensions of aging can be found in gerontology, the academic study of aging and its application to policies and programs.

Even my own field of psychoanalytic psychology has largely ignored the body until the past two decades, which is a shame since Sigmund Freud as a young man well understood the importance of the body as the foundation of the self. He famously said in 1923 that the "ego" (which we now call "self") is "first and foremost a body ego" and that "the ego is ultimately derived from bodily sensations . . . chiefly from those springing from the surface of the body"[9]—an understanding that is being affirmed today by research on touch and on the mind-body connection.

The young Freud also understood a lot about the way that sexual or other trauma could produce bodily symptoms—in fact, all of his first "hysterical" female patients were suffering from *physical* symptoms like paralysis of the hand, tics, leg pain, and so forth. And he knew that these bodily symptoms could be changed or relieved through talking with an empathic listener, like a psychoanalyst, who was trained to get beneath the surface into the feelings and bodily sensations that told the real story.

Unfortunately, Freud's early understanding of the bodily foundation of the self went largely underground as he developed more abstract theories centering on fantasies and conflicts arising solely within the mind. For the next half-century, psychologists behaved as if therapy took place between two minds, the therapist's and the patient's, which each happened to reside in bodies. Body development remained in the shadows, as something that "just happens."

The Body Emerges

Only recently has the body begun to come out of the shadows to receive some of the recognition and investigation it deserves. In the past several decades, something of a revolution has been taking place in the field of psychology—particularly in relational psychotherapy, attachment theory, and trauma theory—as well as in cognitive science, philosophy, sociology, rhetoric, literary theory, feminist and queer cultural studies, and, of course, neuroscience. Scholars from these diverse academic disciplines are suddenly vitally interested in the body and, as I mentioned, are investigating such questions as how we become aware of having a body; how body development is influenced by family, culture, and language; and how we become embodied.

The body is being reimagined as always in flux,[10] and our relationship to our body as dependent on whomever we are relating to, where we happen to live, and our particular moment in history. We feel one way about our body when we are with Shauna and another way when we're with Robin. We feel differently about our body when we are in a small rural town in Kansas than we do at a cocktail party on Fifth Avenue, where extreme thinness is a marker of status. We would have felt differently about our bodies in the time of the Flemish Baroque painter Peter Paul Rubens (1577–1640), when extravagant sizes were celebrated, than we did in the 1950s or do now in the twenty-first century. Studies show that *Playboy* centerfold models, Miss America contestants, female television characters, and models in women's magazines have all gotten thinner and thinner since the 1950s.[11] In other words, the body is not a static body, but something that is heavily influenced by social and cultural forces and always in the process of being reconceived.

In my own arena of what's called "relational" psychotherapy and psychoanalysis, we are becoming more and more body-focused—most particularly when we are working with individuals who have undergone severe trauma, whose traumatic memories are often "stored" in body sensations at the same time that their emotions may be numbed. We now pay attention to our patients' shifting body sensations, as well as our own, and we carefully track how our body responds to the patient's body and how the patient may be responding to our bodily presence. Some of us now view psychotherapy as, in part, a process of bringing the mind and body together, of "mind-body integration"—another way of describing what I have already spoken of as embodiment.

The recent explosion of research and knowledge in the field of neuroscience keeps confirming, revising, and expanding on the insights from psychology. Freud's early insight into the body as the foundation of our sense of self is getting major confirmation from the exciting and evocative findings emerging from the new fields of "brain mapping" and "interoception."

The Body in the Brain

Remember the yoga teachers who changed their bodies and their sense of their bodies through movement and breathing? We now know, by means of new scanning technology, that they were also changing what scientists are calling their brain "body maps."[12] Scientists have shown that when we perform a certain activity with our body, a particular area in the cortex of our brain is activated. If you touch your knee, for example, the sensation is collected by special nerve cell receptors in the skin, funneled into your spinal cord, and sent to a particular place in your brain's cortex. A touch to your head goes to another area in your cortex. Those parts of the body that perform a lot of important, complicated actions, like the hands or the lips, have a larger area of the cortex devoted to the sensations of touch in that part of the body.

Scientists think of the whole body as "mapped" or "encoded" by the brain in this way. They imagine multiple metaphoric "maps" on the brain's surface that link to specific parts of the body and record or encode certain functions. You can imagine this "map" overlaid on the brain's cortex like a picture of your body—fingers, hand, arm, shoulder, neck, chin, lips, nose, and so on. But the map of the fingertips and the mouth and lips will be proportionately larger than they are on your actual body, since these areas need to record more complex sensations and manage more functions.

Our most important sensory map is the touch map, because touch is our most important sense. We can survive without the special senses of vision, hearing, smell, or taste, but we cannot exist without touch. Touch helps us know that we have a body and helps us define the outline and limits of our body, gives us a sense and feel of our body, and protects us from harm. But we have maps for other senses, too, including thermoception (temperature), proprioception (sense of the body's position and motion in space), vestibular (balance, or the sense of up and down), and nociception (pain).

We also have a primary motor map in our brain for making movement. So, for instance, the motor neurons in the muscles of our hand that allow us to move our thumb link through a chain of neurons to a particular area of the cortex. And we have an important visceral map of our insides that gives us access to our internal sensations, many of which we call our emotions. The sensation of tension in our gut—that roiling, cramping feeling—is related to a particular area of our cortex that records that sensation. In short, we now understand that our brain maintains multiple maps of our body's surface and interior, with areas devoted to every swatch of our bodies.

Particularly fascinating is recent research that shows that your brain maps not only the body but the space around your body, called "peripersonal space." Your brain cells keep track of everything and anything that happens within this invisible space, which extends an arm's length around the body. This helps you know where your body is positioned in space and allows you to locate objects approaching your body, like a baseball zooming toward your head. This space actually expands and contracts depending upon your activities. For example, if you're eating, your touch maps will include your fork as an extension of your hand, which allows you to feel the food as if you are touching it with your own body. If you're playing baseball, the bat is annexed as an extension of your arm. If you're making love, your maps expand to include your partner, and your maps and your lover's maps join together in passion! In other words, as the wise have long suspected, the self does not end where our flesh ends but rather blends with the world, including other beings.

Interoception

The most fundamental and fascinating body maps are the "supermaps" of sensations arising from *within your own body*. Internal sensory signals streaming from all over your body get integrated and encoded in a particular part of your brain cortex called the *insula,* which maps the "state" of your whole body. As mentioned, our ability to read and interpret these signals is called *interoception*[13]; it's like a sixth sense you didn't even know you had that, I will argue, can be developed to help you age more successfully. The revolutionary science of interoception, how you sense yourself from within, is a hot new research area, spawning hundreds of new studies over the past decade alone that are upending our centuries-old belief that the brain is an information-processing machine that can be understood apart from the body.

Neuroanatomist Bud Craig[14] and his team have mapped in detail the neuro-anatomical *interoceptive pathways*, which begin with sensory signals from small-nerve fibers (tracking temperature, itch, pain, cardiac signals, respiration, hunger, thirst, and touch) that get funneled into the spinal cord, up through the brain stem, and finally into a deep furrow at the very top of your brain, the insula. Your brain then integrates all this information and gives you not only a sense of the physiological condition of the entire body but, in addition, your core consciousness, your emotional life, even your sense of "self."[15]

The purpose of gathering all this internal information from around the body is the survival of the human organism. This interoceptive process helps you maintain your physiological *homeostasis*, or stable equilibrium, while at the same time consuming the least amount of energy. It gives you a reading of how well you're doing physiologically at any given moment, which you experience as variants of "good" or "bad." You may feel strong or weak, grounded or scattered, vitalized or depleted. New research shows that information coming from your digestive tract is particularly important for monitoring how you're faring overall. You are constantly updating your sense of yourself based on what's going on in your body.

Your brain is taking in important information about your body through another process called proprioception, which refers to your awareness of your body in space—its position, motion, and equilibrium. An example of having good proprioception is being able to throw a ball without having to look at your throwing arm. Your body sense, therefore, includes both your body sensations/emotions (interoception) and your sense of movement (proprioception), which gives you the location, size, and shape of your body. In this book I focus particularly on interoception, because of the proliferation of cutting-edge research in this area and because it is so crucial to our overall sense of well-being, particularly as we age.

Many years ago, when I was in my late twenties, I took myself for a month to an alternative university in the mountains of Colorado. There I was immersed in an intense and intoxicating schedule of classes in Buddhist meditation, poetry, tai chi, and Gestalt therapy, as well as lots of hiking, singing, drumming, drugs, and dancing. The 1970s! While I was grooving on all of this, I was certainly aware of "expanding my consciousness" through exciting new ideas and experiences, taking lots of emotional risks with new friends, and often being outside of my usual comfort zone. But I did not begin to understand how profoundly I was changing until I got home and discovered that, unbeknownst to "me," my usual, familiar body had changed into what felt in certain ways like another body.

I found myself feeling more sexually free with my husband and more sexually attractive in general. I found that I could suddenly dance with an abandon I had never thought possible, and—most shocking to me—my handwriting had changed! When I returned to my grad school classes, I saw that my handwriting had morphed from being cramped and loopy to flowing and not loopy at all. What remains most exciting is that these changes proved to be permanent. It turned out that my experience that summer was not only what we then called "mind-altering" but body-altering as well.

I had learned firsthand how experience can reshape the body and the mind. But it is only in retrospect, as I write this book, that I can begin to understand what happened. I think now that all that meditation and tai chi and dancing must have deepened and integrated my internal, "interoceptive" sense of my body, so I could experience my bodily self with more freedom and joy.

It has been scientifically proven that the body does, in fact, have a mind of its own, as it did for me that summer long ago. Neuroscientists have shown that some 95 percent of what we think takes place outside of conscious awareness, the result of unconscious processes in our brain and body.[16] Even when "we" make decisions, our brain decides moments before "we" do, because our unconscious mind is significantly faster than our conscious mind at processing information. By scanning the brains of participants, for example, scientists at the Max Planck Institute for Human Cognitive and Brain Sciences[17] predict several seconds in advance which hand the participants would choose to press a button.

We've had some inklings of the bodily foundations of the mind since the nineteenth century, beginning with the philosopher Edmund Husserl and the psychologist William James. But most scholars studying intelligence and cognition had, until recently, continued to treat the mind as separate from the body—as if the mind runs on the brain as software runs on the computer. Beginning in the 1990s, however, theories of "embodied cognition"[18] emerged and have since blossomed, to the point where there is now agreement across many fields that the body plays an essential role in cognition. Some have made the radical argument that the structure of thought itself comes from the details of our physical experience—for example, that our early bodily gestures give shape to our later speech qualities, like rhythm or tonality.[19] Most recently, cognitive scientists have begun to include interoception, the sensing of the internal state of the body, in their understanding of social cognition and how people process interactions with other people.[20]

In short, we now know that the experience of our body—the people it touches, the things it feels, the movements it makes, and, especially, its internal sensations—is the primary experience of our mind. As science writers Sandra and Matthew Blakeslee put it, "Nothing truly intelligent is going to develop in a bodiless mainframe. In real life there is no such thing as a disembodied consciousness."[21]

Interoception and Neuroplasticity

Your body maps, created very early in life, are what neuroscientists call "plastic"—that is, they are capable of being constantly reorganized and redrawn in response to experience and practice or bodily injury. When you do planks at the gym to tighten your abs, you're not only strengthening your core, you are also reconfiguring certain body maps in your brain. The more you work your abs, the more you sprout new connections between brain cells and strengthen existing connections, literally increasing the area devoted to abdominal muscle maps. When you do body awareness practices, like yoga, you are literally thickening the insula and beefing up your interoceptive abilities.

Until the 1960s, when Marian Diamond and her colleagues at UC Berkeley began their paradigm-changing research on neuroplasticity,[22] everyone believed that our basic brain geography was set in stone by late adolescence—that the ability to remodel the brain, the brain's "plasticity," was only for kids. We now know that brain structures continue to change for the rest of our lives. The brain is constantly working, adapting our maps minute by minute to changing circumstances, making the experience of embodiment possible and making it feel natural. Your brain will be different when you finish this paragraph, because the brain changes by making or strengthening connections between neurons when you do anything, including reading a sentence or even having a thought!

We've known for decades that if you practice something for a long time, like basketball or the violin, it will result in changes in your brain. But it wasn't until the advent of a new brain scanning technique called functional magnetic resonance imaging (fMRI) in 1990 that scientists could observe brain activation and measure structural change in the brains of living humans. The earliest attempt was the now-famous study of London taxi drivers by Eleanor Maguire and her team.[23] Back before the advent of navigation apps, taxi drivers in London had to study three to four years to memorize the city's 25,000 streets and then constantly rely on their spatial representation abilities to make their way around the city. Maguire's team did two things. They scanned the brains of beginning cabbies and measured the brain region called the hippocampus, which is responsible for spatial representation, then they tested these same cabbies after five years of experience and found that the spatial area was remarkably larger. They also compared the scans of the experienced cabbies with those of London bus drivers and found that the spatial area of the brain was measurably larger in the cabbies than in the bus drivers. Why? Because the bus drivers, who followed the same route every day, didn't need to exercise and develop that part of their brain as much.

How about the *aging* brain? We know that brain volume and neuroplasticity declines in general with age, but the central question for us is whether the brain structure of older adults can change in response to learning or practicing, as the younger brain does. The answer is yes, but not as much. In an important study, Janina Boyke and her team[24] scanned the brains of twenty-five older female and male adults (average age sixty), then taught them to juggle three balls at a time, a novel and challenging task. They then compared the jugglers' initial brain scans with scans taken three months later, after they had gone through intensive juggling training and practice. They found that the amount of gray matter had increased in those areas of the brain important for visual motion as well as several other functions, as a result of the training. What is even more exciting is that Boyke and her team found that the older jugglers showed the *same* kinds of changes in the *same* areas of the brain as a sample of twenty-year-olds they had taught to juggle in a previous study.

And how about those tantalizing reports about actually growing new brain cells, or neurons, in older age, what neuroscientists call *neurogenesis*? While we know that neurogenesis continues to decline throughout our lives after adolescence, numerous rat studies have shown that new brain cells can still be formed into old age, but only in two specific areas of the brain, both in the hippocampus, which is a center of learning and memory and spatial representation. Direct evidence that *humans* can grow new brain cells has remained elusive, however, with major studies recently coming down on both sides of the ongoing debate.

And how changeable or "plastic" are those little "caps," called *telomeres*, that protect the ends of our chromosomes and that get shorter as we age? Every time a cell divides, some of the telomeres get worn down, sending a signal to the cell that it is no longer protected and can die. It is, in fact, the shortening of the telomeres that makes us look and feel older. Biologist Elizabeth Blackburn shared a Nobel Prize for the discovery of telomerase, an enzyme that replenishes and renews the telomeres, but no one has yet found a way to use telomerase to slow human aging.[25]

Blackburn knew that chronic stress accelerates aging and poor health, so she and health psychologist Elissa Epel decided to figure out why and how. How does stress "get under the skin"? They studied the mothers (or other caregivers) of young children with severe chronic disorders, who live day in and day out with the most terrible stress, and they found that chronic stress accelerates the rate of *cellular* aging, shortening telomeres and lowering telomerase. But they also found that *some* of these mothers were able to maintain their telomere length and keep their chromosomes happy. How did they do it? Blackburn and Epel, who later coauthored *The Telomere Effect*,[26] which caused quite a splash, concluded that it has to do with how you "perceive" your stress. If you experience a difficult situation as very stressful, your stress hormone, *cortisol*, rises, which is damaging to your body. If, on the other hand, you see the situation as a "challenge," blood rushes to your heart and brain and energizes you. They concluded that we have more control over our stress than they ever imagined. Not surprisingly, exercise, healthy diet, lowering overall stress, meditation, getting enough sleep, and social connection can also increase telomere length, stimulate neuroplasticity, and improve longevity and health in general.

Embodiment and Brain Change

Although your ability to feel your internal body sensations decreases slightly with age, evidence is mounting that you can heighten your awareness of your internal body sensations with practice. The research on interoceptive awareness has sparked greater respect for Eastern practices like yoga, mindfulness, and tai chi, which have for centuries focused on building body awareness.

This is what happened to neuroscientist Sara Lazar, who switched from studying molecular biology to the science of yoga and meditation after she discovered that yoga, prescribed by her doctor for overuse injuries from running, not only cured her injuries but significantly increased her happiness and quality of life. Her best-known study[27] found that meditation can produce structural alterations in those parts of the brain that control interoceptive ability, memory, executive functioning, emotion regulation, happiness, empathy, and compassion. What surprised her most was the finding that fifty-year-old meditators had as much gray matter in their brains as twenty-five-year-olds, which suggests that meditation and yoga may slow down the *age-related* atrophy of certain parts of the brain controlling memory and executive functioning. In later chapters, we'll look more at the effectiveness of meditation, yoga, and other interoceptive training techniques. We'll also learn how an *impaired* ability to interpret body sensations is implicated in disorders like psychosis, autism, body image disorders, and anorexia.

Tuning up our interoceptive awareness is one of the best things we can do for ourselves. Yet for most of us it's not so easy. The mind still holds sway in most sectors of our Western industrialized society, making it difficult for us to attend to, value, and care for our bodies enough to become truly embodied. Living grounded in our body can become even more difficult as we age. It's hard to feel comfortable with and in our older body if we are deathly afraid of aging and in pitched battle against it. I'll be proposing some strategies to help us end this battle for good.

Chapter 2

Triumphing Over the Body

Hi, You. This is your body. I have a request. I'm sending you messages 24/7 about what you need to feel healthy and happy. My nerves are beaming the latest news from all over me, and my brain is putting it all together to keep you up to speed on how you're doing. Your brain and I are also whipping up emotions to help you figure out what to do with yourself from one moment to the next. Please pay attention!

I work my axons off day and night for you with no vacation. Yet, you rarely think about me. You hardly seem to notice me, although you do spend plenty of time thinking about how I look. Face it, without me you can't survive. Without me, you are nobody. Get it? No body.

Do I really need to remind you? I'm getting older and starting to feel some changes. It's kind of a relief because I don't react so much to things, and I'm actually happier and more chill than I used to be. But I'm not as strong or gritty. My balance isn't as good. More than ever now, I need you to really listen to me, to keep me at my best. When parts of me go wrong, I need you to do whatever it takes to heal me. It doesn't help when you act like I'm the same as I was twenty or thirty years ago. It's not good for me. I really need you with me now, not with some made-up body.

One evening, three friends and I found ourselves talking about aging, and I asked them if I could turn on the tape recorder:

Me: So, how do you all feel about getting older?
Victoria, age seventy-three: I find it shocking, humbling

and . . . sobering. I'm talking about the changes in my body. Because I don't feel that different in terms of flexibility, level of energy, strength. But when I look in the mirror at my body, I just feel really sad. . . . I look at young women in certain kinds of outfits and I think I can't do that anymore, that's over. I used to be able to wear anything. I totally banked on my body and my appearance, more than I realized at the time. Losing that is this kind of loss that is like death. It's over, the absolute end of something. I just can't get over the "forever" of it. . . . All these illusions . . . they're just going.

Me: You're really feeling the loss. Is it helping you to acknowledge it?

Victoria: Hmm, I wish I could say it's bringing me into a different way of being and changing my values [laughing ruefully], but from where I am now, it just really sucks. I wish I had something more wise or spiritual or developmentally appropriate to say, but I would be lying.

Annie, age sixty-seven: A woman came in last week to take my picture for my brochure, and she looked at me for a few seconds, then said, "Boy, what I could do for you!" [Roars of laughter from the group.] She did come back with a nice, well-edited picture of me.

Me: I really do love all your faces at this age. There's much more depth and character and attractiveness too. But I agree that the aging body is harder to make something good out of. We can do a lot with our faces, hair, clothes, but . . . the aging body? Can you make something good out of it?

Connie, age seventy-four: Sometimes I say, this is just the way bodies go. I'm losing my elastin. I can try to make it better with Retin A, or cover it up more, etc., but otherwise I just say, fuck it, I'm gonna do what I want to do and enjoy my husband and my friends and make the most of it!

Me: Some people talk about a different attractiveness in each stage of life, that each age has its particular kind of beauty. Do you think we can get there?

Connie: I can't get there when I go to my dermatologist, and she says, "For $400 I could just fill all this in for you and then your lips will look bigger."

Annie: I don't know. . . . Here I am, a sixty-seven-year-old woman, still obsessed with my weight and my appearance.

Me: Look, there's a huge number of us, 40 million women Boomers alone. We've added thirty years to the average person's life over the last century. This is all new territory. Could we create a different sense of what we're supposed to look like when we're older?

Victoria: What is attractive for evolutionary reasons is symmetry, youth, vitality, health. I don't think this is going to change.

Connie: On the other hand, when we get dressed up, men still respond to us.

Me: Like the guys in the hardware store this afternoon! They loved us! [All laughing.]

Victoria: Yes, but that's with our clothes on.

My interviewee Clarissa, age fifty-five, is part of the next generation, Gen X. Her protest against aging is less conscious and acerbic than those of Victoria, Annie, and Connie, but it's still there in what she said to me:

> I often still feel much younger than my age. In my sense of myself, I'm somewhere between twenty and forty, and I always will be. Sometimes I'm shocked when I look in the mirror, depending on the lighting. Some light is okay and I think, okay, fine, I can identify with that person, then suddenly the lighting is stronger or there's a different angle, and I suddenly feel freaked out about how old I look. It's like I'm looking at someone else.

Are you like Victoria, who's clearly resentful and depressed about aging; or Annie, who's trying to "stay young" by obsessing over her weight and appearance; or Connie, who says, "nothing I can do about it, so, why not just enjoy what I have"; or Clarissa, who's only dimly aware of getting older except for moments when "the light gets brighter"? Or are you more like me, avowedly "pro-age," advocating age acceptance? Except, well . . .

just this morning I decided to go to my medicine cabinet to look at my current and not-so-current skin care products and found . . . hmm . . . Rapid Wrinkle Repair Night Moisturizer, Rapid Wrinkle Repair Serum, Regenerating Cream, Anti-Wrinkle Deep Wrinkle Night Moisturizer, and Ageless Intensives. All these names suggest that something is "broken," causing a "wrinkle" that needs to be "repaired," and that skin can be "regenerated" to make you "ageless." The word "serum," in particular, sounds seriously medical, like something that goes right into your blood.

Do I actually believe that these products can "fix" my wrinkles or "regenerate" my aging skin? I do not. What I believe is that these creams and lotions and serums can slightly and temporarily improve how my skin *looks* by plumping it up or exfoliating the older, duller skin cells. But it's all part of the same thing. Whether we choose these potions, or chemical peels or "sanding," or the knife, it's all about age denial or age shame. I don't want to look my age. I want to "pass" for younger.

In our society, unlike ancient societies or Asia today, younger is better. Younger is more attractive. Younger is also smarter, cooler, more fun, more valuable. Our society is not very interested in older people, especially older women. My eighty-nine-year-old interviewee June told me: "Focus groups or marketing groups don't include anyone over fifty. So, they don't ask us our opinions or market to us. We've fallen off the edge, invisible. People are surprised to find out you're an outspoken, effective human being. They expect doddering, and I've never done that."

When our society acts as if we have nothing to offer, we can internalize this lack of interest and assume we are not very interesting or important. Small wonder that practically all of us want to avoid aging. There are as many ways to push away aging as there are humans in the Western world. Whether we see it as a mild affront, or a big loss, or something so painful it can't even be contemplated, getting older is something none of us looks forward to.

What we are talking about here is *ageism*, a term first coined in 1968 by the world-renowned gerontologist, author, and visionary Robert N. Butler, who championed the rights and needs of older people and became the first director of the National Institute on Aging. Feminist Margaret Cruikshank, another aging expert, says, "We must *learn* to be old. . . . It is not just a natural process like breathing, but something we are initiated into, and we learn to be old partly in response to the ways we are treated. . . . Aging is a creation of this time and place, more cultural than biological."[1] In other words, it is "socially constructed" by the society we grow up in.

Our reluctance to accept the reality of aging is captured in a theory called "the Mask of Aging,"[2] which suggests that we experience age as a mask concealing our more youthful, more authentic self. Age is felt to be a disguise that hides our true feelings, motives, attitudes, and beliefs—in part because our culture's aging stereotypes leave us little room for expressing our unique identities. According to mask theory, we are just seen as "old."

Our culture's particularly destructive "social construction of aging" makes it difficult for us to age comfortably. We are urged to deny aging, defeat aging, or what I call "triumph over aging." We become ageist ourselves. Indeed, ageism appears to be our country's "last socially sanctioned prejudice."[3] It is also the only "ism" directed at ourselves: we see our own future, older self as inferior to our younger self, says Adrienne Applewhite. This creates a strangely disorienting and destructive divide between who we are and who we will become: "Talk about not wanting to belong to any club that would have you as a member! Which would be funnier, and a lot less ironic, if it weren't the club that everyone is counting on getting into."[4]

My aim is not to perform some kind of hocus-pocus to allow you to see the aging of your body as *positive*—hardly a winning proposition—but simply to help you accept its inevitability with some equanimity. This, I believe, is a minimum requirement for aging comfortably. For is it not unfair and self-destructive to rage against the aging of our bodies, when aging is a *universal* fact of life, an integral part of our human life span (if we're lucky)?

The Enduring Sexism of Ageism

When we add sexism to ageism, it becomes a double whammy for women. Women, much more than men, are the targets of our society's ageism, and we internalize the general disdain for aging women as our own shame. We feel compelled to learn the "art of aging gracefully"—a phrase that I remember actually liking a few decades ago but now infuriates me. Why should we have to age "gracefully," which, in this case, means something like "without showing it"? "Gracefully" is a word reserved for women if there ever was one. Yes, we want to age in ways that help us feel (and look) as good and healthy as possible, but "gracefully"? Gracefully for whom? Men, of course. So, we keep on "remodeling" ourselves so we never ever "look our age" or "act our age."

Just look at the "funny" greeting cards women send to one another. They're all about being alcoholic or sex-crazed and blithely unrepentant—a kind of pathetic attempt to suggest that we're all still wild and crazy. Humor, as Freud said, is one way of managing anxiety. Nora Ephron said it best (or worst) in *I Feel Bad About My Neck*:

> Oh the necks. There are chicken necks. There are turkey-gobbler necks. There are elephant necks. There are necks with wattles and necks with creases that are on the verge of becoming wattles. There are scrawny necks and fat necks, loose necks, crepey necks. . . . You have to cut open a redwood tree to see how old it is, but you wouldn't have to if it had a neck.[5]

Or how about the "eccentric" older "woman in purple" and often feathers, who, even though she may feel sexually "invisible," can at least compel peoples' attention by looking "interesting"?

It used to be even worse for women, as we well know from our childhoods. Think of Simone de Beauvoir's grim, groundbreaking 1949 feminist study of the subordination of women under patriarchy, *The Second Sex*. She was one of the first to shine a light on the female body—how women learn to "live" their own bodies through the hungry eyes of men, rather than from within—and she trenchantly concludes that "to lose confidence in one's body is to lose confidence in oneself."[6] As I've mentioned, brain scans have confirmed Beauvoir's insight: if we are not rooted in our bodies, we cannot be emotionally grounded in ourselves. In her equally grim and exhaustive 1970 study of aging, *The Coming of Age*, Beauvoir again concludes that, as men see it, "a woman's purpose in life is to be an erotic object. When she grows old and ugly, she loses the place allotted to her in society: she become a Monstrum that excites revulsion and even dread. . . . She becomes an other."[7]

Shortly thereafter, Susan Sontag argued in a definitive 1972 essay, "The Double Standard of Aging" (which I still remember reading and rereading), that beauty for women is identified with youthfulness, meaning that women become "sexually ineligible" much earlier than men.[8] The male gaze, Sontag suggests, focuses on the imperfections, including the aging, of our female bodies, not our minds or spirits. Women then internalize the male derision of older women and end up full of self-hatred.

To be with an aging woman reminds men of their own aging and their own terror of aging, particularly of their loss of virility. Men traditionally turn to younger women to quell these terrors. It is also true that feelings of self-denigration and shame are often intensified for those who were once beautiful, like Victoria at the top of this chapter. Consider this passage from Sigrid Nunez's 2020 novel *What Are You Going Through*, which is all about aging: "I remember, the elderly and once beautiful woman said, after I reached a certain age it was like a bad dream—one of those nightmares where for some reason no one you know recognizes you anymore. . . . I'd never been in the position of having to work at making people like and admire me. Suddenly I was all shy and socially awkward."[9]

We must also admit that certain things *have* gotten better in recent years. Not only do we have full-size models in women's clothing ads but we have "older" models—probably around age fifty. There are also some much older actresses, like Jane Fonda (born 1937) and Lily Tomlin (born 1939), who play best friends on the TV show *Grace and Frankie* and appear together on the talk-show circuit lauding the joys of female friendship in older age, with which I fervently concur. Judi Dench (born 1934) and Helen Mirren (born 1945) are also famous and popular older actresses. *Our Lives at Night*, starring Robert Redford and Jane Fonda playing shy lovers in their seventies, is one of the sweetest little movies ever made. In the fashion world, Eileen Fisher (born 1950) brought compelling fashion to women in their forties and up, and now Swedish designer Gudrun Sjoden (born 1941) aims even older, with some white-haired models age sixty and over. All of these women, of course, are still the exceptions.

So then, we must ask: With increasing acceptance of older women as actors and models—as "attractive" women—and with so much more inclusivity in our society for all colors, creeds, ethnicities, and sexual orientations, why are we of the older generations *still* so defiant when it comes to aging?

The Anti-Aging Generation

Why is it that we—younger and older Boomers alike—seem to be even more rejecting of aging than *previous* generations? Why are we so obsessed with "beating" aging that we buy millions of books on age-reversal and support a multi-billion-dollar cosmetic, fitness, surgical, and pharmaceutical anti-aging industry? Among our cohort in modern American culture, the drive to deny and defy aging just seems to be increasing.

It has a lot to do with when and how we grew up, says author Susan Jacoby.[10] In her perfectly titled book, *Never Say Die: The Myth and Marketing of the New Old Age*, she posits that the unparalleled prosperity of the post–World War II society in which we grew up and became young adults set us up to believe that we would always be able to get what we wanted. A combination of postwar economic expansion, the GI Bill, mortgage rates of 4 percent, and other factors led to a period of unprecedented prosperity and upward class mobility. Our parents took the heritage of the New Deal for granted, and so did we. I remember, in the middle-class neighborhood of Evanston, Illinois, where I grew up, seeing family after family in which a man with a middling salary, maybe $10,000 a year at that point, could buy a home and a car and support a wife and four children and send those children to college and have money left over for vacations and a good savings plan.

When we Boomers started coming of age in the late 1960s, we expected more of the same—at least those of us in the least impoverished strata of society. Economic prosperity, we assumed, was the new norm. This assumption, Jacoby writes, "bred a careless confidence about the long-term future that has influenced our approach to every stage of our lives and has been shaken only in recent years."[11] "Careless confidence" was me, stopping my work in journalism in the mid-1970s to travel to India, to write freelance articles on sexism, and make videotapes on the women's movement with a group of friends. Money? Who me, worry? We expected that there would be plenty of jobs waiting for us after we had realized our human potential. A new period of life called "youth" was conceptualized by author Christopher Lasch: "youth" was what you now were until age thirty.[12] All of this was understandable, given our early beginnings, but there were also some serious consequences of this overly optimistic, free-form period. Many of us, including Michelle and Barack Obama, made very consequential decisions to delay child-rearing until the last minute, and some found ourselves scrambling to overcome infertility as we passed age thirty-five, a mistake not made so frequently by members of the next generation.

The Boomers' belief that there will always be enough to go around has led to two other foundational Boomer expectations, according to Jacoby: first is faith in the possibility of repeated self-transformation through self-help, whether it be through psychotherapy, spiritual transformation, or cosmetic surgery. This belief in reinvention is key to our mentality. The second flows from the first and is our trust in the capacity of medicine and technology to transform the process of growing old when self-help efforts fall short. Indeed, our belief in self-transformation, coupled with the women's movement, has radically opened up the world for many of us, allowing us to move beyond limiting or self-negating views of ourselves and to expand our educational, career, social, and travel horizons beyond anything our parents could have imagined. But Jacoby's main point here is that our belief in self-transformation, especially through medicine and technology, may help explain why so many Boomers act as if we can also defeat aging.

There are many fascinating advances in the scientific pipelines that could slightly increase longevity—including increasing telomere length, purging senescent cells, reprogramming gene expression, and strengthening the immune system.[13] Yet, most of this research primarily offers better maintenance and repair of the body, not a "reversal" or even a major deceleration of aging. And scientists do not now believe that we will ever find a single elixir of youth, because every body is different, with its own unique biology, genetic background, and environmental exposure.

In short, we cannot overturn our body's general plan for us; we can't turn back the clock.

At the same time, we do know a lot about how to make the most out of our older years—by building our body awareness, emotion regulation, and attentional capacity through meditation and other forms of mindful attention, and by exercising our bodies and brains, eating right, and maintaining supportive relationships. If we take good care of ourselves, it is now very possible for most of us to remain strong and healthy into our eighties or even nineties. It is also true that how "old" we feel or act is very individual and depends greatly on our cultural and family expectations.

We also have to acknowledge the role of *stigma* in how we feel about our declining bodies. The stigma against disability of any kind is still very much alive in our society, causing many people with disabilities to try to hide or override their infirmities. Ageism combines with stigma to create shame in older people about "looking old." Many refuse to use wheelchairs or walkers because the stigma is so great—even if it means never getting out of the house![14] I've noticed that many older people are using high-tech walking sticks (which read "athleticism") rather than canes (which read "disability"), and that we prefer Apple watches or Fitbits (which read "hip"), rather than medical alert bracelets or necklaces (which read "elderly"), to monitor and report falls. Only about 20 percent of people who would benefit from a hearing aid actually wear one, even though uncorrected hearing loss can triple the risk of falling and is linked to depression and dementia.[15]

So many tributaries have flowed together to create our current ageist society, including our media-saturated obsession with youth; the unprecedented prosperity and optimism of our generation's early lives; our belief in our ability to endlessly reinvent ourselves through psychology, science, and technology; and the stigma of disability. Small wonder that books like *Stop Aging Now! The Ultimate Plan for Staying Young and Reversing the Aging Process*, by Jean Carper, and *Aging Backwards*, by Miranda Emde-White, continue to sell thousands of copies. But really . . . stop aging now? Stay young? Reverse the aging process? I don't think so! These books may help us lead healthier and happier lifestyles, but they are not going to stop us from getting older.

This certainly does not mean that we should focus only on our vulnerabilities as we age. We want to live vibrantly and enthusiastically and be strong and feisty in the face of physical challenges and proud of ourselves when we overcome them. My point is simply that our sanest choice is to see our aging body as it actually *is*, rather than how we wish it were or how it used to be, to develop a better relationship with our *actual* older body. We must stop trying to find solutions to the "problem" of aging, as if it were a disorder.

Triumphing Over the Body

Our fantasied drive to defeat aging is just one manifestation of a much broader cultural problem, which I call the "triumphing over the body" narrative. This narrative requires an active overriding of the body's needs, as well as the recruitment of unconscious defenses, like my interviewee Clarissa's denial. The triumphing over the body narrative spawns the mind-body disconnect I spoke of in chapter 1, a societal split that valorizes our *conceptual* self-awareness over our bodily self-awareness.

Listen to my sixty-one-year-old patient Diana, who struggles with excruciating lower back pain. "My body? It's better if I just don't think about it too much, because then I get depressed, so I just white-knuckle it. I just blast through the pain. I don't let it get me down." She feels proud that she is so "strong," and she tells me that her family and friends really admire her for overriding her body and not letting her pain get in the way of her athletic activities. Our society does too. It is filled with narratives of women (and men) trying to conquer their bodies—like Olympic superstar gymnast Simone Biles, who pushed herself almost to the breaking point at the Tokyo 2021 Summer Games, or Oprah Winfrey, conquering her weight "problem" (again). We will, of course, always admire athletes and other people who strive to do the best they can and expand the limits of what we thought humanly possible. But an elite athlete must also be utterly in tune with her body and utterly respectful of the specific needs and vulnerabilities of her particular body so she can take excellent care of it during training and not injure it in competition. This is the opposite of "overriding" the body—although athletes, like everyone, can sometimes lose their wits and go too far.

How about you? Do you engage in extreme diets? Do you work till you drop day after day? Do you "forget to eat" all day and feel proud that you may have lost a pound, even though you're lightheaded from low blood sugar? Do you pride yourself on being able to function on five hours of sleep? Every one of these activities is self-defeating and has been proven by science to be bad for you. Most likely, you already know this and do it anyway. However, each of these behaviors is a slap in your mortal face. The attitude that "I can do what I want to my body and it will be fine"—"I" am stronger than my body—reveals that strange, fantasied distance between mind and body, as if one could actually separate the two.

Seventy-five-year-old interviewee Dierdre, who was a professional dancer in her twenties, told me:

> The hardest part for me is being kind to my aging body. I want to be able to force my body to do the things I used to be able to do without consequences. Running, jumping, leaping . . . the joy of movement. Riding my bicycle as fast as I could down a hill, like flying. My body was an instrument I could use. It was at my command. There was a oneness between my desire and my body responding. Now, the desire is there, the body is there, but getting the two together is the problem these days. I have trouble taking good care of my body because I want it at my command as it used to be. I know what I should do is stop and listen to it and say, um, okay, I need to do a little horizontal meditation for a while. But it's really hard for me to let up.

Women's "triumph" narratives so often have to do with the body. The ongoing epidemic of eating disorders among (mostly) women in our country is a quintessential example of women trying to subjugate their bodies in order to look and feel forever youthful. While older women are not typically as actively anorexic or bulimic as younger ones, a large proportion continues to severely restrict food intake, overeat compulsively, or alternate between the two. And there's another concerning new body-triumphing trend: people are replacing aging joints with bionic parts at younger and younger ages in order to continue doing taxing sports like expert skiing, surfing, or marathon running, at older and older ages. The percentage of hip and knee replacements performed on men and women starting around age forty-five has rapidly increased over the past decade.[16]

"Triumphing over the body" is a particularly bad narrative for us as we age. It's not a good idea to override, ignore, or abuse our bodies at the very time that they are becoming more vulnerable and need more attention and intervention. In fact, ignoring our body prevents us from doing all the things that would make us feel better. The goal of positive aging is to stay *healthy*, not young. Denial or protest or "triumphing over" our aging bodies does not make us feel better. It does not support us. It does not strengthen us. Fighting aging is a way of rejecting ourselves, telling ourselves we're not good enough. Not letting ourselves age is a way of not letting ourselves *live*.

Triumphing Over Death

At bottom, of course, our fear, disgust, or anger at the aging body is really about our fear of death. The body is the harbinger, the bellwether, the messenger of our mortality: "As we age, we look towards death, and we look away," writes psychiatrist Calvin Colarusso, an expert on adult development. "As we move inexorably closer to death, it becomes harder to deny its inevitability."[17]

Let's return for a moment to Clarissa, age fifty-five, who, you remember, suddenly saw herself in a certain light in her mirror as older than she thinks of herself. As my interview with Clarissa continued, something very interesting happened, as she realized she's not only seeing her*self* in that mirror. She says:

> I'm also looking at my older sister who I can really see aging because I don't see her very often. And I can see glimpses of my mother too, who actually . . . oh . . . this is so interesting! . . . My mother died when she was fifty-five, my age now, so I always anticipated that this year would be so intense for me, and then I forgot about it until this moment. I haven't been thinking about it,

not even on my fifty-fifth birthday a month ago, until just now with you. . . . I feel creeped out. There's so much about my mother's body . . . my body came from her body. . . . Does my body look like her body? At some point in her fifty-fifth year, my mother didn't have a body, her body was done. Can one "outlive" one's mother?

In this very moving moment, Clarissa not only acknowledges her fear of getting older but also her fear of dying as her mother did at a young age—a fear so profound that she remembers, then forgets, then remembers again that her mother died at the very age she is now. We can see how her fear of aging slides right into her fear of death and denial of death. Clarissa finds herself looking toward death, then looking away.

In his famous 1973 book *The Denial of Death*, Ernest Becker suggests that consciousness of death is the primary repression—not sexuality, as Freud thought—and that the "terror of death" is a primary motivator of human activity: "The idea of death, the fear of it, haunts the human animal like nothing else: it is a mainspring of human activity—activity designed largely to avoid the fatality of death, to overcome it by denying in some way that it is the final destiny for man."[18]

Freud, at age fifty-nine, personifies the denial of death in the character of "the poet" in his 1916 essay "On Transience": "No! it is impossible that all this loveliness of Nature and Art, of the world of our sensations and of the world outside, will really fade away into nothing. It would be too senseless and too presumptuous to believe it. Somehow or other this loveliness must be able to persist and to escape all the powers of destruction."[19] Freud calls this attitude "a revolt . . . against mourning."

So, when portents of our mortality arise, we try to kill the messenger, which is never a good idea. The news brought by the messenger arrives anyway. And if we kill the messenger, we can't learn all that she has to tell us about the feared event ahead. It is much better to work with the messenger, learn everything you can from the messenger, to better prepare for the message of our impending mortality.

The sages agree: the anticipation of death, which informs the later stages of life, leads to a narcissistic crisis. How we respond to this challenge determines in large part how well we will do in our final life stage.

In this and the next chapter, I will encourage you to try to look mortality directly in the eye. A true encounter with our own mortality allows us to see into and acknowledge reality in a way that was not before possible.

My friend Maureen said it best: *"Aging is like a straight shot of reality."*

Triumphing Over Nature

For centuries now, we have used the Earth for our own pleasure or expediency, soiling and overheating our precious planet, our only home. Now, we can finally, starkly, see its desecration. As I wrote this chapter in September 2020, I was still "sheltering" in my home, not only from COVID-19 but from dangerously unhealthy air caused by massive wildfires fueled by parched grasses and wind currents caused by climate change. A few days earlier, when a thick layer of ash hovered over northern California, blotting out the sun and turning our blue sky an unearthly orange, it seemed that our earthly home might be gone forever, and I was plunged into grief.

Despite twenty-first-century science, we can still think like medieval theologians, imagining ourselves masters of the universe, bending natural processes to our will. In truth, of course, we are simply a part of nature, like every other animal, bird, insect, or tree. Indeed, if you count the one hundred trillion microbes in our guts, only 10 percent of the cells on (or in) the human body are actually human! We hang in the web of nature. Each of us comes into being, ages for a time, then dies. We can't triumph over ourselves.

It makes it so much worse when we try.

Strategies for Rewriting the Triumphing Narratives

How, then, do we begin to upend these narratives of defying, defeating, or "triumphing over" aging/death/nature—which are, of course, doomed to failure? It is imperative that we confront these pervasive societal fantasies of overturning the natural order, because they ravage our bodies, our peace of mind, other living beings, and our planet. These narratives make our older years a time of struggle and unhappiness when, in fact, they can be a time of unprecedented freedom and joy.

How can we stand up to the din of fake anti-aging news that strafes us from every corner? Here are some strategies to help us more comfortably accept the reality of aging while, at the same time, continuing to live with purpose, vibrancy, and joy. These suggestions, of course, are not equally important for everyone or every age group.

Strategy 1: Engage with Aging

Some people want to sleep through aging, but this is not a good idea. As we move into older age, we need to be *awake* to what's happening in our bodies and minds, and not only because it helps us take loving care of ourselves. We don't want to miss our own aging process, because it's such a vitally important stage of our life, with a new kind of happiness, aliveness, and equanimity and so much to be learned and enjoyed, which I describe more in the rest of the book.

I urge you to seek out and take advantage of the myriad resources on aging out there—books, articles, podcasts, interviews, documentaries, blogs—and to be sure to see the few good movies or TV shows with aging characters. I also find it so useful to talk honestly with my husband, friends, and relatives about the ups and down of getting older. Why do so many of us feel we have to be alone with it or hide it or act as if it's not happening to us? Sharing our experiences of getting older with others helps us be more honest with ourselves. It's a fool's game to deny what's actually going on.

My interviewee Katrina, age fifty-nine, doesn't want to miss a thing when it comes to the aging of her body: "I actually have a 'practice' of acceptance of my aging body. I look at my naked body in the bathroom mirror, like when I'm coming out of the bath. It helps me to know what my body looks like naked. It helps to have a reality check. When I stare at myself in the mirror, I have to accept my older body." As William James said, "My experience is what I agree to attend to."[20] We can't nurture or change what we have not experienced. I'm sure it's no secret by now that I decided to write this book partly because I wanted to be more awake to my own aging, so I could age better myself.

As we age, we move through new life stages, from middle age to "young" old age (roughly our sixties and seventies) and "old" old age (roughly eighty and above)—just as children move into the teenage stage, then into the young adult stage. As younger people, we tend to look forward to the next stage, which comes loaded with new opportunities, challenges, and pleasures. So why, as older people, do we strive to stop ourselves from continuing through the next stages, which are just as distinct and full of new opportunities and challenges (albeit not all welcome ones) as our earlier stages? It's folly, is it not, to refuse to inhabit a life stage that is ours, a stage where our body clearly reveals the truth even while our mind may try to deny it?

Truly engaging with aging requires us to be honest and open with ourselves. Hedda Bolgar, a psychoanalyst and political activist, said in a film interview when she was ninety-seven: "I live by one idea now, which is that . . . we don't try to avoid things, we don't try to hide things. We are committed to uncovering things and dealing with it. And I think that needs to be true of the relationship with the patient and it needs to be true of how you live and it needs to be true in every way."[21] Bolgar died six years later when she was 103, old enough to have attended Sigmund Freud's lectures in Vienna. She was still seeing patients and teaching until a few days before she died.

Hedda Bolgar was extraordinary. But it is also true that there is something about aging that allows many of us to finally lay our cards on the table, to not "hide" any longer. As James Baldwin said: "Not everything that is faced can be changed, but nothing can be changed until it is faced."[22] When we have nothing to hide and can age without shame, we find there is not much left to triumph over. It is this openness to ourselves, flaws and all, that can make us increasingly able to age with authenticity and honesty. We are more simply human. We can let go of how our body should be, how life should be, who we think we are. We can ask: Who are we if not this younger body, this familiar story? By really paying attention to our aging body and mind, we can wake up to who we are *now*.

My seventy-four-year-old interviewee Elizabeth (whom you met in chapter 1) told me how she woke up (literally) to being older: "I had a dream, not a dream with a plot or a story line, but more of an internal, maybe verbal, realization. I'd been reading this book about Epicurus and how he thought old age was the pinnacle of life. So, in the dream, I'm thinking, 'Okay, now I'm here at this older age of seventy-four.' My heart hurt a little—I thought, how sad—but at the same time it felt *real*."

Strategy 2: Ride with Change

Flexibility is always singled out by aging experts as one of the psychological characteristics that helps us age more comfortably. Those who stay the healthiest and live the longest, research shows, somehow manage to adjust and adapt to the physical, mental, and emotional changes that come with aging. My seventy-eight-year-old interviewee Carey is a great example of adaptability. She reflected with me on the many changes she's had over the years:

> I got a diagnosis of osteoporosis early in my forties, but I forestalled it for many years by taking estrogen, calcium, etc. I didn't think about it a whole lot. But then I started having changes in my balance, and I had several serious falls, one requiring surgery. And now, some arthritis in my hip. I've really had to change how I walk through the world—literally. I used to move around quickly, and now I have to go slowly and carefully. I don't like it!
>
> That's when I realized no one was going to stop the train of aging, so I better take my seat on the train 'cause that's the train I'm on. I better learn to enjoy the ride as much as I can. I had to give up Zumba and do balance exercises, which I absolutely hate. Then I found something that's actually enjoyable and that's tai chi, which I do with a lovely group of older people in the park. Is it my favorite thing in the world? No. But it really helps my balance and makes me feel more graceful.
>
> I've also been trying to shift my thinking toward my body, this miracle that's carried me to the age of seventy-eight. It's like I have this old beloved car that's in the shop a lot, and I have to maintain it more than I'd like, but I devote myself to it because I'm grateful for it.

We have to keep adapting and growing. I have an old friend with a bad knee who could no longer run, and she took up hiking. Then when hiking was no longer possible, she took up swimming. When her vision dimmed, she took up audio books. As Mary Pipher says in her book on aging, "If we don't grow bigger, we can grow bitter."[23]

We can also ride with the changes of aging more easily if we distinguish between those things we can change and those we cannot. You can't, for example, expect your short-term memory to be as good as it once was, but you can enjoy your heightened ability to make connections among ideas from different parts and levels of your brain. You can expect to plump up your biceps by lifting weights, but all the triceps exercises in the world won't tighten that pendulous flesh of your upper arm.

To be maximally flexible, it makes sense to "travel light."[24] It helps to unload ideas of ourselves from the past that no longer apply to our new stage of life. Do I still have to be the quickest, most clever person in the room? Do I still have to get men to notice me on the street? Do I still have to whizz around getting a ridiculous number of things done in order to feel like a valuable human being? Aging requires letting go, which always involves a bit of mourning.

Here, I must evoke that central Buddhist teaching called "impermanence" (*anicca* in Sanskrit). Everything, *everything*, is always changing. Nothing is permanent or solid. "Impermanence" does not refer only to the changing of the seasons, our moods, or politics. At the most profound level, it means that everything we love and treasure—including our partners, children, parents, friends, even our self and our Earth—will not only keep on changing and transforming but will eventually pass away. Everything comes into being, and everything passes away. To try to "triumph over" that truth brings disappointment, frustration, and defeat. The only approach to life that can ultimately bring peace is to accept the way things really are—that things are constantly changing.

It is here that *aging* is the best teacher of all, because we can really *see* the changes in the crinkling and sagging of our flesh. Of course, we've been aging in a steady, programmed, predictable way since we were born, but it gets so much more *obvious* as we age. The process of change is all laid out for us to see with our own eyes—if we let ourselves look.

Aging is like a straight shot of reality.

Strategy 3: Zoom Out

The writer May Sarton, beloved for her wise and unvarnished daily journals of her later years, writes in her book *At Seventy*, "The trouble is that old age is not interesting until one gets there, a foreign country with an unknown language to the young, and even to the middle-aged."[25] And older age is more than just "not interesting"—for so many, it is something to be feared and avoided. As a result, many of us, of all ages, don't really let ourselves *see* the older people around us, or we see them as "not me." We don't really pay attention to them.

I asked my interviewee Molly, age sixty-nine, how she felt about getting older, and she said:

> As I get older, I've got a different perspective. It's like a camera pulling back so my field of vision gets broader, so I can see myself and the relative importance and lack of importance of things in my life. I never really understood that advice before about putting the big stones in the jar first and then putting the little ones around them. But now I don't have trouble telling them apart. Not to say that there aren't changes that impede this bigger vision, like fear of falling, fear of losing my mental acuity, fear of being alone. . . . I guess maybe it's really just a trading of fears; when you're younger, there's this painful anxiety about so many things, but as you get older there's a kind of fatalism that can be very helpful. Hardly anything feels catastrophic anymore.

It helps tremendously to "zoom out" on our lives and take a wider view of our life span from birth until death. And we can take an even longer perspective if we add in the life spans of loved ones whose lives we lived with them. My "life span" then goes back 130 years to the birth of my beloved grandmother, who I called Nonny, born in 1882, in Dayton, Ohio. She knew the Wright brothers, who owned a bicycle shop a few blocks from where she grew up.

Taking a lifetime perspective, we can see that we are getting older from the moment we are born until the moment we die. We don't suddenly step over an invisible boundary into a new country called Old Age, where we are suddenly required to wear orthopedic shoes. Aging is an integral part of adult development. It is a building process, an accretion of experience, growth, and learning, not a crisis. Feeling "old" is a state of mind. Some people feel it when they're fifty, some when they're eighty-nine, and some never. In fact, if we think of older age as running from sixty to one hundred (forty years), the sheer variety of people in that age span is huge—more heterogeneous than any other life "stage."

From this broader, life-span perspective, we can look ahead as well as back and can spend time trying to *prepare* ourselves for the years to come, whether it's middle age or older age. One way is to purposely spend time around people older than ourselves: we'll find that some seem quite different from us in certain ways, while others seem a lot like us. Just as there is no country for old men (or women), there is no prototypical older person. A particularly useful exercise, suggested by aging author Anne Karpf,[26] is to try to *see older people as our future selves*—to see them not as foreign or separate, but simply as how we too will be, as we continue along our natural human life course.

Strategy 4: Look Mortality in the Eye

Most people who grew up in Western societies are terrified of death, to the point where they cannot let themselves contemplate it, much less ask their lawyers to write up their wills. As Woody Allen said, "I'm not afraid of death. I just don't want to be there when it happens." Even the word "death" is suffused with fear, dark colors, melancholy, deep organ chords, and the grim solemnity of funeral rites. Death is dramatized; it's not quite real. By denying our mortality, we create an unconscious and delusional belief in our immortality.

In Buddhist thinking, Death is one of "the Four Messengers" whom Prince Siddhartha (later to become the Buddha) encountered when he first explored the world outside his sheltered and privileged life behind the palace gates.[27] The messengers (who also include Aging and Sickness) are teachings—harbingers of the reality we all have to face. The awakening of the mind to old age and death occurs when one realizes at a gut level that these realities are actually going to happen to *us*, not only to other people. The Buddha even sent his followers out to the charnel grounds to contemplate the state and decomposition of the dead body as a first step toward imagining the state and decomposition of one's own dead body. The Buddha was teaching impermanence: one cannot triumph over aging and death. For Buddhists, the meditation on death is the supreme meditation.

In the books by Carlos Castaneda, who had millions of us aflutter in the 1970s, the fictionalized Mexican sorcerer Don Juan had a similar wise message. "Death is our eternal companion," he said. "It is always to our left, an arm's length behind us. Death is the only wise adviser that a warrior has."[28] Castaneda came to experience death as a palpable entity, a fleeting shadow that he could perceive out of the corner of his eye, a presence that gave him a certain sobriety, courage, and humility, in contrast to the "drunken," death-denying strutting of people from the Western world from which he came.

Accepting that our life will eventually end—which scholars call "finitude" or "transience"—is the most important emotional task of the last third of life. Keeping mortality in our peripheral vision, like Castaneda, gives us courage and humility and emotional depth. It also frees up tremendous energy that we've been using to maintain all of our defenses against acknowledging aging. Knowing that death can come at any moment can allow us to live life to the fullest.

Strategy 5: Work with Your Fears

Unfortunately, it is not so easy to look ahead to the end of our life or accept our aging body just as it is. As my friend Victoria lamented at the beginning of this chapter, losing her lovely young body was "a kind of loss that is like death." If we truly stop and reflect on our aging body, we are likely to feel some combination of fear, disbelief, anger, embarrassment, sadness, and loss, which can then activate our "triumphing over" narratives. It is most helpful if we can identify, admit to, and acknowledge these darker feelings as they arise and let ourselves feel them as fully and fearlessly as we can. When difficult things are experienced honestly and openly, they become much less overwhelming. Walking into the lion's den increases our courage and confidence.

Let's consider *fear*. Specific fears will vary from one woman to another, but the underlying anxieties are so often the same, revolving around loss, helplessness, and isolation. When I asked my interviewee Julie, who is sixty-eight, if she had fears of aging, she nodded forcefully and said, "Oh yeah!" and told me that recently she'd been feeling fear a lot whenever she felt a sharp pain in her knee. "It freaked me out," she said, "because the pain seemed to be getting worse, and I'm afraid I'll end up in a wheelchair." I asked her if she would be willing to tell me about how she worked with her fear. "What helped me most," she said, "was using RAIN." (RAIN is an exercise developed by meditation teacher Tara Brach; the acronym stands for *Recognize, Allow, Investigate, Nurture.*[29]) "First," Julie said,

> I let myself *recognize* the feelings and feel them as much as I could. Then I tried to get hold of the thoughts that were freaking me out, like "I'm not going to be able to hike anymore, and I'll need a cane or maybe a walking stick." Then, it started to get really crazy, and I started thinking, "I won't be able to walk and I'll be stuck at home.... This is it, the beginning of the end!" I felt devastated, but I decided to move on and do the second step and *allow* this whole experience to just be there, just as it is. I found my body was so tense I was jumping out of my skin, so I got up and got some pretzels and tried to *allow* the fear again, and it was a little better this time. So, then I moved on to *investigate* it and get curious about it, and it got really, really interesting, in an awful kind of way. This picture of my Aunt Louise just rose up in my mind, sitting there in her wheelchair when I was a young kid, and I think—not sure I'm remembering this right—that one time she had fallen out of her wheelchair or something.... Then I went to the last step, *nurture*. I put my hands over my heart and said compassionate things to myself in a really kind voice. I tried to think about what I needed to feel better, and I realized I needed to "get it" that I'm not Aunt Louise, and I needed reassurance that I can heal this knee and that I can get help healing it. I don't have to simply put up with it and become isolated.

Julie had been aware that her catastrophic thinking was creating and maintaining her fear, but she hadn't been able to get a handle on her fear until she started working with it in a focused, deliberate way. In my experience, the RAIN exercise, which can be found online, is very helpful, and I would add another step that I have found useful: after you have identified your particular fear, and the thoughts and sensations that go with it, "rub" your consciousness up against the fear and ask yourself questions like, What does it feel like? Does it have a texture, a shape? In other words, really get to know the "feel" of the fear in both your body and mind. When we work with our fear in these ways, we see that fear is not concrete and real, but, rather, a series of thoughts, accompanied by physical sensations. Realizing this, we sometimes find that the fear miraculously dissolves, and we're left simply with sensations . . . and then nothing.

As we get older, it is important to try to get a handle on our fear, because some older people can get so lost in their fears that life becomes hell. It may be reassuring to learn that many people who have been through disabling illnesses report that the *fear* of losing one's bodily functioning, particularly one's mind, is much worse than the disabling event itself.[30]

Embarrassment about aging is another problem for most of us at one time or another, particularly since embarrassment is, well, so embarrassing. I was recently working as a consultant to a young therapist on her psychotherapy case, and when I stood up to say good-bye at the end of the session, I suddenly pitched headlong to the floor at her feet! Unaware that my right foot had gone "to sleep," I had stepped on it and felt nothing there to step on. And, while this could happen to anyone at any age, my first thought was how it made me look feeble, debilitated, out of control—that is, *old*. My consultee's reaction was worried and solicitous, offering to call a doctor and stay with me, but I said, "No, no, I'm having lunch now with a colleague who can help" (which was true) and cheerfully got her out of my office as quickly as I could, even though I was in severe pain and had, in fact, badly sprained my ankle!

Whether we're struggling with fear or embarrassment, anger, disappointment, disbelief, sadness, or grief, it helps to become aware of and begin to work with these feelings sooner rather than later, so that when things do get more difficult with age, we're familiar with these darker states and already "in practice" working with them.

Strategy 6: Trust Your Body

The brain, when unmoored from body sensation, is in the business of worrying or fantasizing about an unknowable future. Our anti-aging "triumphing narratives" are stories cooked up by our tricky, often misguided brains to quell our fears about getting older. This is why it is so important to consult and listen to your body. Your body is designed to keep you safe, healthy, and in balance, and you need to let it do its job. You can hurt or even permanently damage your body if you try to "triumph over" it. Indeed, once you've developed more body awareness, it feels downright self-destructive to ignore, "override," or mistreat your one precious body. Only your body knows what's real for you, because only your body can *sense* what you need and who you really are. Getting comfortable in your body, therefore, is one of the best ways to calm your fears of aging.

The body has its own ways of knowing, its own profound wisdom. When I asked Clarissa, for example, what she found most surprising about being older, she said: "The way my body is telling me I'm getting older even though I'm still feeling younger. Like having to stretch when I get out of bed in the morning. I know it's really changing. It's really happening." Clarissa is discovering that her body's communications are more trustworthy than those of her mind. I will share much more about how to tune in to, trust, accept, and inhabit your body in the chapters that follow.

Strategy 7: Mourn Your Losses

Aging leads not only to unwelcome changes in body and mind but also to an accelerating march of loved ones passing away. Losing people in our intimate circles is inordinately painful and saddening, and the longer we live, the more the losses can pile up. I watched my mother, who lived to be ninety-four, lose every single one of her six siblings and old friends.

The waning of our capacity to have certain treasured *experiences* is another kind of distressing loss. My husband, due to arthritis, has lost the ability to downhill ski, and now, because of arthritis combined with the travel limitations of COVID-19, worries that he will never again scuba dive, which has been an incomparably blissful experience for him.

Similarly, when I asked my interviewee Diana how she felt about getting older, she said:

> I'm scared about aging. I don't like it—partly because I had my children late. I think if my children were older, I might feel a little more at peace. But at sixty-seven, with a twenty-four-year-old and a thirty-year-old daughter, I'm aware there may be lots of things I won't be around for, like seeing grandchildren grow up. How are things going to turn out for them? The world is so complicated right now; I wonder how they'll be doing when I'm not there.

Whatever losses come our way, it is imperative that we let ourselves mourn them. Many of us fear that the grieving process will be a bottomless pit of suffering we won't be able to climb out of, so we try to distance ourselves from the magnitude of our feelings. Actually, we're better served by doing the very opposite. Letting ourselves deeply feel our loss, as painful as it is, allows us to feel more connected to ourselves and more alive, which allows us to heal and move on more quickly. When we let ourselves grieve, we also deepen our compassion for ourselves, for others who are grieving, and for the grief of the world, and we find ourselves more moved to help.

A few years ago, I did a weekend workshop on aging with the revered Buddhist teacher Anna Douglas, then eighty years old, who made the interesting suggestion that we begin now to work with the "small deaths" related to aging to help us prepare for the final, big one. For example, we retire from a job, give up waterskiing, or our kids move out of state. Douglas suggests going to the "gym of compassion" for each of these "small deaths" to strengthen the muscle that can deal with loss. This builds confidence. Start with 2-pound weights, she says, and, after a time, you can handle a 500-pound weight. Bringing compassion to yourself for each loss is key. She ended the exercise by asking, "What if you could simply relax at the moment of the 'big death'"?

You'll learn basic loving kindness meditation in chapter 6, a practice in which we bring compassion to ourselves. You may wonder why I am referencing Buddhist thinking so much in this chapter. It's quite simple.

Buddhism is the most helpful belief system that I'm aware of for accepting change, shedding defenses against unwelcome truths, and being with what *is*. In short, it can help us accept aging.

At this point some of you may be wondering why anyone would want to accept the inevitability of aging if it comes with loss and mourning and intimations of mortality. Maybe the idea of taking a more defiant, placard-carrying stance—"Beat Aging!" "Forever Young!"—sounds a lot more attractive and upbeat. And yes, it can feel that way. All I can say is that if denying and defying aging really worked, I would be all for it. The problem is that it *never* works to hide from reality. It takes enormous energy to keep those defenses propped up against the ever-mounting evidence of aging, and all that energy goes toward pushing away rather than living life to its fullest. "I remember how much trouble my poor mother had with aging," Molly told me, "because my dad wanted a younger woman. My mom felt she had had something, and now it was lost. She loved her grandchildren, but she didn't want to be a grandmother, because that meant she was old." Molly's suffering mother could not accept who she was. When we do not accept our age, like Molly's mother, we cannot accept who we *are*. We can't fully inhabit our bodies or live in the present. Because we are not "all there," we cannot feel grounded or truly alive. It's only when we learn to age comfortably and positively that we can *live* well as vibrant older women.

Strategy 8: Let New Identities Arise

Let's not forget that change goes in both directions: it not only brings wear and tear and loss but also new beginnings. We may find ourselves shedding old pieces of our identity as we age and then just as naturally creating new ones to replace what we have lost. My friend Margo is now seriously pursuing songwriting. Dorty is avidly writing poetry. I used to be much more social—or thought I was supposed to be—while in recent years I find myself craving more solitude, more empty space in which I can just be. I used to feel I had to widen my professional community by getting to know the movers and shakers, while now I'm mainly drawn toward being with close friends and family. I sense this has something to do with my feeling more comfortable being in my body and in the present moment. My decision to write this book for a general audience certainly emerged out of aging—I found myself wanting to write woman to woman, as *me*, in my real, everyday voice, rather than from a professional vantage point. Sometimes, new identities are famously created by taking up challenging new activities at advanced ages, like Grandma Moses, who started painting in earnest at the age of seventy-eight, or Julia Hawkins, who took up running at the age of one hundred and ran the 100-meter dash in 39.62 seconds at the age of 101.

My interviewee and friend Nancy, who had worked in high-level social service jobs all her life, decided at the age of fifty-eight to move with her husband to a beautiful rural area of a developing country in Latin America. They soon found themselves getting to know and love the indigenous people who lived nearby in a small jungle community of three hundred. Over the years, they have spearheaded building a small medical clinic, a little factory to produce cleaner wood-burning stoves, a childcare center, a school, a ball court, and a community center—all funded through donations and all now run by the people themselves. "Seeing this community thrive makes us so unbelievably happy," Nancy says. "I'd rather be here than anywhere else."

We are always works in progress. This doesn't change just because we're over fifty. We can keep *adding* abilities, qualities, resources, and activities and offering our gifts to the world. We feel ourselves enlarged rather than diminished by aging. To help you think more about what you've lost, what you've gained, and what you still have to offer, now and in the future, I'd like to offer an exercise focused on how our body experience, even our body identity, changes as we age, prompted by an exercise on aging from Zen teacher Lewis Richmond.[31]

Self-Guided Exercise:
Changes in My Body Experience/Identity

Ask yourself this question: In the past three, five, ten, or twenty years, what aspects of my body experience have changed? Take some time to let yourself muse on the following questions, feeling your way into your body and thinking deeply about how your body and your body sense may have shifted over the years. If it helps, take notes.

- Changes in my appearance (body shape, posture, muscles, skin, face, hair, etc.)?

- Changes in my gait?

- Changes in the "feel" of my body?

- Changes in my body due to injury or illness?

- Changes in my physical activity? (For example, doing less, doing things more slowly, not being able to do things I used to do.) Explain.

Now switch to the positive side: What new aspects of my physical identity have I created to replace what I may have lost?

- Have I added new physical activities or modified existing ones?

- Do I have a different sense of my body? A different relationship with my body?

- Do I pay more attention to my body? In what ways?

- Do I take better care of my body? In what ways?

- Am I more accepting of my body? In what ways?

- Do I feel a certain pride in my body just as it is?

- Can I imagine new possibilities for invigorating my body experience or body self that I have not yet tried or put into practice?

To help you fully grasp the importance of your body in determining who and how you are, I now want to explore how the body, including its maps in the brain, is "made"—how it develops and comes alive mainly through relationship, starting in the womb. What determines how your particular body will live in the world and what kind of relationship you will have with your body? What is your inside story?

Chapter 3

The "Making" of the Body

When Judith was growing up, her mother would become frantic with fear whenever Judith left home. Her mother worried that Judith would fall down and hurt herself, eat something that would make her sick, or get bitten by insects or rats. Her mother was particularly fearful that her daughter would get abducted. So, Judith never went out of the city to walk in nature or to the ocean to swim, and she never played any sports outside of gym class. Even riding a bicycle or ice-skating was considered too dangerous. Now, at the age of sixty, Judith is a very smart and attractive but underachieving woman. She has a glaze of weariness and defeat. To this day, she is afraid of doing anything athletic or even exerting herself for fear of tiring herself out, which she believes will cause her to get sick. She is afraid of falling. She suffers from dizziness, fatigue, and various kinds of gastric distress.

You know you have a body and that it is like no one else's. You may think of it as frail, attractive, heavy, agile, ugly, strong, defective, shapely, funny-looking, sexy, energetic, skinny, clumsy, or invisible. But you probably haven't given much thought, if any, to how your body came to be the way it is, how you came to sense and feel it, and how you came to think of it as "my body" and part of "me." For most of us, our body just *is*. We think it developed according to some innate blueprint, some pre-programmed process.

But that's not how it works. The fact is that your body sense—as well as, to some extent, your actual physical body—must be "constructed" slowly over time through countless interactions with your parents and other caregivers and with your culture. Your body self is constantly being created and shaped by what's happening to you and how you interpret these events. And it takes a very long time, if ever, to develop a sense of really "living" in your body, being "embodied."

It is critically important, as you get older, to understand more about how your body sense became what it is today. Why? Because you can't remodel something until you know how it was constructed. In this chapter I explore how your sense of your body and, to some degree, your actual body was forged in relationship. I'll be focusing mainly on infancy and early childhood, but also looking at adolescence, menopause, and later life. Many of the processes by which your body was "made" in your early years are the same ones that you can now use to revise and "remake" your body as you get older.

Shaping Your Body Sense in the Early Years

Your first experience of relationship is bodily. In the womb, the sensory world of your mother's body *is* the world: the smoothness of her uterine walls, the wetness of her amniotic fluid, the sounds of her heartbeat, breathing, and digestion, and the rocking of her ongoing movements. After birth, your caregivers' love and care continue to be communicated primarily through bodily contact, and it is these bodily interactions that help create and mold your sense of your little body.

I briefly described *interoception* in chapter 1—that is, how your body-mind develops through the sensing and processing of internal sensations, which give you a reading on the "state" of your body, how regulated you are physiologically and emotionally. In fact, hunger signals from our gut provide our very earliest information about what is good and bad in the world. The catch is that when you're a newborn, your immature body can't move around enough to generate all of the necessary sensory signals to create this internal sense of yourself. You need your caregivers to do some of it *for* you. Aikaterini Fotopoulou, a creative young neuroscientist and psychoanalyst, contends that from the very beginning of life, you need to interact with your caregivers in specific bodily ways in order to activate your own interoceptive abilities. Your mental representation of "my body" (which translates to "me") that gets built up in your brain actually *includes* your mother's body. How your mother interacts with your body is experienced by you as *sensing your own body*. In short, your ability to sense yourself from within and maintain your internal equilibrium is completely dependent on embodied interactions with another person. "The bodily and social origins of the self appear as tightly interwoven," Fotopoulou says.[1]

Let's now explore five especially important ways that caregivers shape your sense of your body. These processes are particularly crucial during infancy and early childhood, when your body is developing at breakneck speed and is almost completely dependent on your caregivers, but they continue to be important throughout your life.

Touch

Our skin, which most of us think of simply as a covering for the rest of us, is actually our largest organ, and it is our primary body-sensing organ. Touch is the first sense to come online, and our caregivers' touch is absolutely essential for our development. Holding, patting, stroking, jiggling, wiping, squeezing, kissing, rocking, nuzzling—these are not only ways our mother (and other caregivers) communicates with us emotionally, but the means by which our sense of our own body and our own self develops.

There is a particular *kind* of touch—slow, gentle touch—that is now believed by Fotopoulou and others to be essential for interoception.[2] There are special receptors in what is called the "c-tactile" system of the body that respond only to stroking in a soft, gentle manner. It used to be believed that this "affective touch" system was only operant in more primitive mammals, but now it turns out that man and beast are the same in terms of affective touch. (But you already knew that about your cat!) Being lightly stroked by another person is very calming, and it helps you create a sense of your whole body and maintain your internal equilibrium. It can even down-regulate your experience of pain. Affective touch even shows you something about the emotions and thoughts of your caregivers.

Affective touch appears to be uniquely important for solidifying the boundaries of your self—that is, helping you psychologically "separate" yourself from others and develop the feeling of "owning" your own body. A famous experimental setup, the Rubber Hand Illusion (RHI)[3], reveals the powerful connection between affective touch and body ownership. You can try it at home with a friend:

Place a rubber mannequin's hand on a table, facing away from you, palm down, and then lay your real hand palm down next to it, making sure both hands are in the identical orientation. Then place a cardboard partition between the two hands, hiding your real hand but leaving the fake one in plain view. Have a friend sit across from you at the table and gently stroke both your real hand and the rubber hand with a feather in exactly the same way and in the same rhythm. Soon, if you are like most people, you will feel those sensations coming from the false hand, which now feels like a part of your body!

The illusion works because synchronous visual and tactile information come together in combined vision and touch maps at the back of the parietal lobe of your brain. But what's relevant here is that the illusion works best when slow, gentle stroking, or "affective touch," is used, because this kind of touch is particularly effective in increasing *interoception*, your ability to sense your internal body sensations. The RHI also proves again how malleable, or "plastic," your body sense is. It's also fascinating that people show different degrees of ability to experience this illusion. Those who are most adept have been found to have greater body awareness. Anorexic individuals, who have low sensory awareness, are "immune" to the Rubber Hand Illusion.

Sometimes, when the baby and her caregivers are interacting bodily, they feel in perfect synchrony, promoting moments of "fusion," and sometimes these embodied interactions lead to inevitable moments of asynchrony, when the baby experiences self-other distinction. Through the back-and-forth between synchrony and asynchrony, you come to experience yourself as a distinct human being.[4] These bodily interactions with caregivers also help you experience a sense of *agency*—the ability to take action on your own. When your mother helps you do things—like turning you over or holding you up so you can see out the window—she's letting you feel like you're doing these things yourself. Your mother's actions and reactions generate changes in your own interoceptive states, ultimately helping you build up a sense of being an effective human being. People who have not received enough affective touch as infants and children, research shows, are more likely to experience anxiety, depression, and addictions later in life.

As I have delved deeper into the latest neuroscience on touch, I've been excited to discover how much of it was anticipated by some of our greatest psychoanalytic theorists. Freud, as mentioned, initially conceptualized the ego (now "self") as "first and foremost a body ego" and believed that "the ego is ultimately derived from bodily sensations . . . chiefly from those springing from the surface of the body."[5] In other words, our *skin*. Today, we might say that the self is first and foremost a body-being-touched-and-held-by-another self and that the healthy development of the self is powerfully affected by the quality of the touch we receive as infants.

The great psychoanalyst Donald Winnicott most dramatically envisioned the new science of body development, particularly interoception, when he wrote about what he called the "psychesoma" to emphasize that our psyche and soma cannot be separated:

> I suppose the word psyche here means *the imaginative elaboration of somatic parts, feelings and functions,* that is, of physical aliveness. We know that this imaginative elaboration is dependent on the existence and the healthy functioning of the brain, especially certain parts of it. The psyche is not, however, felt by the individual to be localized in the brain, or indeed to be localized anywhere.
>
> Gradually the psyche and the soma aspects of the growing person become involved in a process of mutual interrelation . . . at an early stage of development. At a later stage the live body, with an inside and an outside, is felt by the individual to form the core for the imaginative self with its limits.[6]

Winnicott's "psychesoma" is an integration of body feelings and functions, which becomes our sense of core self. Sound familiar? It is only when development goes awry, he explained, that we feel like "we" are located only in our head, rather than in our whole body. We identify with our thinking function, not with our embodied experience. Mental functioning becomes "a thing in itself," by means of which we try to take care of ourselves when our caretakers are inadequate. Winnicott continued this trailblazing line of inquiry when he later wrote about how we gradually come to experience ourselves as residing in our whole body—what he called the "indwelling of the psyche in the soma,"[7] or being "at one" with the whole body. This is what we now call *embodiment*.

Other psychoanalysts elaborated quite poetically on the power of touch in early development, describing, for example, how the baby develops a "psychic skin"[8] (an amalgam of the baby's skin and her responsive mother), which holds together parts of the developing self on its way toward integration. The infant's experience of her skin being stroked, another theorist suggests, provides the first inklings of a rudimentary sense of self, the "skin self."[9] The baby imagines that she and her mother are located on either side of her skin, and that they "share" it. Because the skin is both "me" and "not me," the baby learns that she has an inside and an outside and that there are boundaries between herself and others.

Psychoanalyst Wilfred Bion's groundbreaking ideas about how the mother or other caregivers "contain" the overwhelming emotions of the baby[10] also anticipated the new neuroscientific findings on social interoception. If the baby is upset, Bion explained, the mother or other caregiver must be able to feel the baby's upset and urgency *in her own body*. In this way, the baby senses that his distress has been received and is being "held" by the mother. This is soothing for the baby. When the mother's body resonates with the baby's distress, she gets a more accurate reading of the nature and level of the baby's distress, so she can respond quite intuitively—deciding, for example, that her infant is hungry and quickly producing her breast. It is this rapid and accurate-enough response from our mother that helps us build an embodied self that feels competent and effective. We learn that we can get people to respond, that we can get help and make things happen. Each of these psychoanalytic theories, once considered metaphorical or imaginative descriptions of mother-child relations, are turning out to be more biologically accurate than we could ever have imagined.

A plethora of exciting new research on touch proves how important physical contact is, not only in our early years but for our emotional well-being throughout our lives.[11] Affirmative touch provides us with a sense of ease and security in our bodies and feelings of being valued and loved. Touch raises the level of oxytocin, an important social-bonding hormone in both mothers and babies. Oxytocin lowers cortisol, a stress hormone, producing feelings of contentment and security. The right kind of touch can lower blood pressure and heart rate. Touch is also the primary language of compassion; if we are suffering, a hand on our shoulder or a warm hug can make all the difference.

Touch can even make the difference between whether a baby lives or dies. Colombian neonatologists Edgar Rey and Hector Martinez, who were working in an underequipped hospital in Bogota in the late 1980s, reported stunning evidence of the importance of touch.[12] Faced with a shortage of incubators for premature babies, these doctors quite serendipitously found that placing the baby high on a parent's bare tummy for several hours a day, with its ear near the parent's heart, reduced the mortality rate from 70 to 40 percent! "Kangarooing," as this practice has come to be known, has been widely adopted, and skin-to-skin holding between parents and preemies for several hours a day is now commonplace in neonatal centers throughout the world. Babies who kangaroo have more stable heart rates, more regular breathing, longer periods of sleep, more rapid weight gain, and faster brain development.[13]

Mirroring

A second crucial process for body self–development is "mirroring"—that is, interactions with caregivers or others that offer the child a *reflection* of her developing self. A parent's face is the baby's first mirror. When the baby looks into her parent's face, does she see a reflection of *herself*? When she laughs, does her parent laugh? Does the baby see the parent's delight and love and admiration? Or does the baby see in the parent's face the *parent's* own mood or preoccupation or blankness? If the baby does not see her babbling, cooing, laughing self reflected back, then she cannot develop a sense of who she *is*; she cannot come to know her true self or true body.[14] Our parents' admiring and loving gaze makes our bodies feel not only loved and beautiful but *real*, as something that really exists.

As the baby develops, does the parent continue to respond with delight to each new body achievement: rolling over, raising the head, creeping, crawling, standing, walking? A child whose physical actions are met with joy and pride will develop confidence and pleasure in her body.[15] The ages of three through six or so—what Freud called the Oedipal period—are particularly important for the making of the body self. Both girls and boys enter a new phase of development in which they want to exhibit and show off their bodies. They are suddenly more competitive and flirtatious. They might become swaggering or seductive, strutting their stuff. How their parents respond makes all the difference. Can the parents enjoy, engage with, and feel proud of their child's new developmental accomplishment? Or do the parents become shocked or worried or disapproving as they observe their child becoming less sweet, innocent, or childlike and try to shut down this important new stage of body experimentation?

It turns out that the kind of response we get as a baby and child to our different body displays and body states determines much of what will get included in our sense of our body and our self. This process of inclusion/exclusion is really quite simple: those behaviors or emotions that are responded to positively by our caregivers get built in; those that elicit a negative response or nonresponse do not. Behaviors and emotions that are not rewarded get shunted off to the side and hidden away in the dark corners of our minds and may become sources of shame or conflict for the rest of our lives.[16]

So why do some behaviors and mental states get a positive reaction and others a negative one? This depends on the parents' expectations and dreams for their child, expectations that can form while the baby is still in the womb or even before conception! Does Mom, who really does not want to pass on her family history of depression, react with delight when her little girl is happily dancing around but become anxious if her daughter seems quiet or sad and then frantically try to stimulate her into liveliness? If so, the little girl will feel like she's doing something wrong every time she feels sad, and she will create a false presentation, revving up her body to appear lively and cheery at all times.

Imitation

Another crucial way that the body gets "built" is through imitation. Because of a paradigm-changing discovery a couple of decades ago, we know a great deal more about how this process works. I'm referring to the serendipitous discovery by neurophysiologist Giacomo Rizzolatti and his team in Parma, Italy, of a new class of brain cells that underlies imitative processes in ways we never imagined.[17] The researchers were tracking what happens in monkeys' brains when the monkeys stretched out their arms to reach for peanuts, and they noted that every time the monkeys made this movement, a specific group of cells fired in the front part of the brain. Then one day, another scientist came into the laboratory and picked up one of the peanuts and—lo and behold!—the researchers noticed that the same bunch of cells fired when the monkeys *saw* the visiting scientist pick up a peanut. It was as if the monkeys were performing the same action themselves, even though they had not touched the peanut! The experimenters had discovered that the brain has a built-in imitative capacity, and they named these special brain cells "mirror neurons." The discovery of mirror neurons is now heralded as one of the most important discoveries about the brain of all time and is the focus of numerous research projects around the world.

Scientists have since replicated these findings in humans, including babies.[18] It has become clear that an infant observing movements is imitating them in his mind—and building them into the structure of his brain—even before he has the capacity to move. His brain is thus being prepared for movement! Mirror neurons actually kick in within minutes of birth. If you stick out your tongue in front of a new baby, he may stick his out, too. So much of what we learn—from word formation, to eating, to walking, to brushing teeth—we learn through our mirror neuron system. Then we spend years, of course, practicing and building into our bodies and brains what we have learned. Mirror neurons may also underlie emotional capacities like empathy, which we explore more in the next chapter.

Movement

A half-century of rat studies has shown that rats thrive when they can run around in varied and stimulating "enriched" environments.[19] And a great deal of subsequent research shows that the same holds true for human babies and toddlers, who need to be able to move freely and frequently for their bodies and brains to develop properly. Fortunate is the child whose caregivers encourage lots of free play and who run, dance, play catch, or climb with him. We need lots of early practice. Movement is crucial not only for motor development but for creating a healthy brain and body sense as well. Repetition is key. We understand that elite athletes, like Steph Curry, have to practice those long shots over and over and over, but it's also true that we all have to practice our parallel parking, dicing the zucchini, or putting on eyeliner.

Actions that are repeated get built into the brain and are reflected in the relative size of our brain's body maps, with larger areas of the cortex devoted to actions that are repeated more frequently. Psychologists have found that this is true for human interactions as well. The parent-infant *interaction process itself* gets built into the brain and becomes part of who we are.[20] For example, if a mother rocks her baby when he cries and repeats this interaction over and over, this soothing mother-infant action sequence becomes part of the infant's memory and sense of self—which is to say, mapped in his insula—and, over time, it becomes part of the infant's ability to soothe himself.

It has also become clear that the brain literally cannot develop without the body sensations that come from movement. In a now-famous study,[21] two kittens were harnessed to a carousel for the first few weeks of their lives; one kitten could walk, but the other had to lie passively in a basket, propelled by its sibling's locomotion. Both kittens had perfectly good eyes and received the same visual stimulation, but the passive kitten became functionally blind! It had no depth perception, couldn't recognize objects, and was unable to navigate its way around a room. Without self-generated movement, the kitten could not give meaning to the unintelligible blobs of visual information coming in through its eyes, and its visual system could not properly develop.

Another fascinating example of the importance of repeated early movement for body development comes from Mali.[22] Because people in

Mali believe that babies with (what we consider normal) crooked legs are unattractive, Malian mothers stretch and exercise their babies' leg muscles with a firm stroking motion. They also hold their babies upside down by their ankles. They do all this repeatedly for months on end. The result? Malian babies are able to walk at around six or seven months old, earlier than babies anywhere else in the world.

We can find a less happy example closer to home, which reveals what happens when babies are *not* able to move freely during a critical early period for body development. Remember all those babies placed in Romanian and Russian orphanages after the Soviet Union collapsed in 1989, who were later adopted by American families? Many of these babies had been kept two or three to a crib, and, because there were not enough caregivers, they received little attention or snuggles. Many were tied to cribs or chairs to prevent injury. Most had lived a year or two in these orphanages. How have they fared? Seth Pollak, a psychologist at the University of Wisconsin, has studied over 150 of these babies and found that they were two to three standard deviations below the norm on measures of motor development, a huge deficit.[23] Only 1 percent of the world's population would be expected to score that low. For example, as they aged they had severe balance problems: when asked to stand on one foot, they toppled over, and their balance did not improve with time.

The Parent's Embodiment

There is also something much more difficult to observe, and less often discussed, that powerfully impacts our body development. Our parent—particularly our mother if we are female—continually transmits her own feelings about her body to us, just as she passes on her fears or talents. Our bodies, like our minds, take their cues from the bodies we grow up with, which themselves express the habits of bodies in the surrounding culture. Does our mother feel at one with her body, or does she experience her body as alienated or hated? If our mother feels uncomfortable about her size or shape or skin color or gender or sexuality or desirability, we'll instinctively "know" about it and may absorb some of her unhappy feelings about her body and develop a troubled body image of our own.[24]

Susie Orbach, the author of *Fat Is a Feminist Issue*, and her colleagues have recently created a powerful, in-depth clinical interview format, the Body Observational Diagnostic Interview (the BODI),[25] to explore what they call the "intergenerational transmission of embodiment," that is, how our mother passed down to us information about how "at home" and comfortable she feels in her body. If, for example, we see our mother anxiously looking at herself in mirrors and store windows and constantly "fixing" her hair and adjusting her posture, we wordlessly learn that bodies need to be constantly fretted about, altered, and "perfected," and we may start worrying and obsessing about our own bodies. Like sponges, we can absorb these unspoken communications from our mothers or other family members or surrounding culture and make them our own.

I now return to Judith, whom you met at the beginning of the chapter. When I first met her in her gray stucco cottage in Oakland, my eyes were immediately drawn to her hands. One hand was almost constantly squeezing the other—apparently a nervous, yet soothing, habit of long standing. She didn't seem to be able to make herself comfortable on the sofa, and she kept worrying about whether I was okay. Was I comfortable in my chair? Was I chilly? Could I hear her well enough?

During our interview, her words were eloquent but seemed almost rehearsed, as if she had told her story, at least to herself, many times before. Judith grew up in a brownstone in Brooklyn. No yard, very few parks. Her brothers played stickball in the streets, but she, being a girl, was expected to stay indoors with her mother and do women's things like cooking and cleaning and, for some reason, constantly dusting all of the framed family photographs. Judith stopped at this point, looked me squarely in the eyes, and slowly shook her head. She went on to say that her mother was always frightened when she had to go out into the world to do errands or go to the bank. "My most vivid memory is her lying on her bed all day with a sleep mask over her eyes during the 'curse.'"

At this juncture, Judith leaned back against the brindle-tweed couch, shut her eyes, and fiercely clamped her lips together. "My mother was always frantically worried about me, afraid I'd get hurt or sick or tired or carried away by some strange man. Every time I left home, I knew she was there at home, imagining me lying in some ditch, dead. My mother never let me go out and play with other kids, and sports were all too dangerous, even bike riding." Judith does have some happy memories of going with her father to the community pool, but she was never taught how to swim.

Now, at sixty, Judith is a talented and attractive but clearly depressed woman who retracts from expressing the fullness of her being. She remains afraid of physically exerting herself, because it might be "too much" for her, and she might get exhausted or ill. She experiences frequent dizziness, eczema, and various intestinal problems.

How might we explain Judith's troubles? We could say that she is anxious or insecure, or, in contemporary psychological language, dysregulated. Or in medical terms, she might be suspected to be suffering from compromised immune function. However, it might be most informative to talk about her *body*. We could say that her body self is unstable and uncertain and that she has received from her mother an intergenerational transmission of body dis-ease. She lacks a healthy sense of her body.

But that is not the end of the story. Judith tells me that, since our interview, she has signed up for private lessons with a therapeutically trained yoga teacher, which she is finding a "revelation."

Body Image Versus Body Sense

If we are lucky, and our body and body sense have been constructed well enough through the processes I've been describing, we find ourselves with a generally positive and stable *body image*, which I will take up later in my discussion of experiencing our bodies "from the inside out." I'll say just a word here about body image and how it's different from, as well as related to, *body sense*. *Body sense*, which I focus on in this book, refers to how we actually feel and experience our flesh-and-blood body. *Body image*, which appears between twenty-five and thirty-six months of age when we first recognize our image in the mirror, refers to the imagined body—how we visualize and experience our body in our mind's eye and how we imagine it in the eyes of others. It is also true, of course, that body sense and body image are powerfully related and that a strong body sense is a major determinant of an accurate and stable body image. Without a well-developed body sense, our body image will not feel real and connected up with our full being and will be more of an abstract, and often inaccurate, idea of who we are. In contrast, a stable and positive body image "fits like a comfortable suit," says psychologist Elizabeth Halsted. "We wear it without being preoccupied by it."[26]

"Remaking" the Body over the Life Span

As you continue to travel through your particular life in your particular body, there are certain times when your body asserts itself more dramatically, calling new attention to itself and jolting and disorienting your sense of your body and your self. These times are adolescence, menopause, and older age. During these particular life stages, your family and cultural/subcultural beliefs can *magnify* the striking physical transformations of the body and render them particularly fraught.

Every family and every subculture broadcasts, or more subtly communicates, their attitudes toward the body. Perhaps you were raised in a strict, religious family, where the body was not to be talked about, or was talked about only with embarrassment or shame. This prohibition on body discussions undoubtedly included sexual behavior and sexual body parts, and it may also have included menstruation, or even pregnancy. In contrast, you may have been raised in an environment where your parents let "everything hang out," as in the communes of the 1960s and 1970s, where people walked around naked in front of children.

Or perhaps weight was a central issue in your family. Maybe you were raised in an area of the country, like "coastal elite" cities, where you "could never be too thin or too rich." Or you were raised in the heartland or small-town America, where having a more plentiful body was the norm, and you were dismayed when you discovered that in other subcultures, your heavier body was looked at with disapproval.

Does any of this sound familiar? Girls and women with negative body images, research shows, have so often had parents who disapproved of or were disappointed by their daughters' appearance.[27] My colleague in the eating disorders field, Ann Kearney-Cooke, found that parents of eight-year-olds who were unhappy with their *own* bodies tended to be more focused on controlling their children's eating and weight. And a recent, particularly unnerving survey of 361 childcare workers[28] showed that a quarter of them had heard children as young as three years old criticizing their own appearance, and almost half had heard ten-year-olds making negative statements about their bodies.

Or perhaps it was the case in your family that women were routinely treated as second-class citizens. One of my interviewees was required to serve dinner to her brother and clear his dishes away. You may have been treated as less intelligent, less strong, or less important than men, or as "ditsy," "eye candy," or "too emotional." Chances are that you internalized certain misogynistic views and began to carry them in your body—by acting ditsy (remember comedian George Burns's sidekick wife, Gracie Allen?) or being overly sexy to please men, or by disempowering yourself by slouching, keeping your eyes lowered, or speaking in a quiet voice.

The amount of physical affection also differs greatly from family to family. Did you get to sit in Mom or Dad's lap . . . or not? Did family members hug or kiss each other or give back rubs? When someone was really upset, did family members hold and comfort that person?

Then there's body care. Your body may have been something to be carefully taken care of through good hygiene, exercise, and regular doctor and dental visits, or it might have been something to be taken for granted or ignored. Perhaps, in your family, it was considered "strong" or even heroic to override the needs of your body even when you were tired or sick or injured. Or maybe—the other extreme—physical health was something to be worried about and obsessed over.

You may have contended with significant bodily difficulty. Maybe you had to manage physical disability or a chronic illness or disorder for some part or all of your life. Or you may have experienced trauma to your body, such as serious injury, surgery, or abuse. Or perhaps you were unable to take care of your body adequately because of poverty or other limiting or stressful aspects of your home environment. My point here is that the life of the body is much harder for some than others—and this, of course, affects our whole sense of being.

Let's look more specifically at those three life stages—adolescence, menopause, and older age—when the body moves front and center and takes a leading role in your life and how you experience yourself.

Adolescence

In your early teen years, your body suddenly morphs into a startling new form, featuring breasts and pubic hair, and becomes almost unrecognizable even to yourself. At the same time, your brain is going through its own high jinx. In early adolescence, as in early childhood, the tiny branches of your brain cells suddenly begin to multiply wildly as part of a normal process of overproduction or "exuberance."[29] These new neural pathways open up myriad new options in your young life. But then, before you reach age twenty, your brain "prunes" about 10 percent of its gray matter, preparing you to specialize in certain areas rather than others. During this reconfiguration, the brain is more vulnerable and easily wounded, making it a particularly bad time for drugs and alcohol. Indeed, the frontal lobe of your brain, which controls planning, organization, and judgment, is one of the last areas to stabilize, not reaching some measure of maturity until your mid-twenties.

As you develop and your body begins to look and feel more like your mother's, and especially if your mother's experience of her body veers toward the negative, your heightened identification with her can lead to having a troubled body sense or body image of your own. Or, if you identified more with your father and he has a problematic body sense or if he sexualizes or fails to admire you, or if your body development skews away from the cultural norm, you can also develop a weakened body sense or body image. You may have trouble experiencing your body sensations or imagining your body in a positive way. Not surprisingly, adolescence is the most vulnerable period for the development of body dissatisfaction and related problems like eating disorders.

Maybe your body developed early, and you reacted by wearing sweatshirts to school to hide your breasts. Or you developed late and suddenly found yourself "uncool" and invisible, because the faster-developing girls were suddenly the popular and exciting ones. Perhaps you had serious dysmenorrhea, which put you out of commission for about a third of the time, and, to make matters worse, you got blamed for being "out of sorts" when you were already in all that pain and discomfort. Maybe you were one of the too-numerous girls who got so disturbed about your weight that you decided to restrict your food intake, or overeat, or throw up what you did eat, and you suddenly found yourself in the deadly grip of an eating disorder, out of control of your own body.

Your new sexuality may have felt to you like a naughty secret, or something you could use to get love or shock and to push away your parents. You might have felt bad about yourself because you had too much sex with too many people, or you might have felt embarrassed or inferior because you had too little sex or no sex at all. Or when you wanted to wear the latest, "cool," skimpy top or dress, your parents may have responded with outrage, disapproval, or even disgust. My interviewee Dorothy had this to say about what it was like in her particular family with her particular body:

> I've had a long, long battle with my body. When I went to boarding school for high school, I started to gain weight and it made my parents really crazed. It made them crazy! It was bad. I got grounded if I didn't eat right. I got lectures about it. My father walked in once when I was coming out of the shower at around sixteen, and he made me put a towel around me and stand on a scale, and then he berated me for what felt like forever. It was humiliating and horrible. And the idea that I was not conventionally pretty was really disturbing to my mom. This was not "the plan." My mother was raised in the 1950s to be good-looking and marry well. That was it. She was a local beauty queen, and my aunt's picture was on tourist postcards. Appearance was everything.

No matter how the world around you responded to your body, one thing is true for everyone: your body after puberty was profoundly different than it was before. Whether you felt betrayed by its changes, or thrilled by its womanly transformations, you basically had a new body. And this body is the one you took with you into adulthood, the one you had through college and your first job, the one that saw you through relationships or not, and perhaps into parenthood. This was who you were as time passed, and then, some thirty years later, things began to change again.

Perimenopause and Menopause

There is a second big resurgence of the body in perimenopause, when it demands attention through wacky menstrual cycles, expanding midlines, night sweats, headaches, mental fuzziness, irritability, insomnia, and so forth. Our primary female hormones, estrogen and progesterone, are waning, as is the male hormone testosterone, which helps us feel strong and sexual.

On the long journey to menopause, life as we know it feels thrown into disarray. It makes us question ourselves in ways we haven't since . . . adolescence. We can feel strangely unfamiliar to ourselves, often making us question the meaningfulness of our work, our activities, our marriage or romantic partnership, or how we've been relating to family and friends. The emotional meaning of losing our fertility, sexual allure, and ability to have children—our very raison d'etre in the eyes of nature—brings feelings of sadness and identity confusion. "Who am I now that my body is different?" Indeed, the risk for depression is an astonishing fourteen times higher than normal for the two years before menopause.[30]

But this is decidedly not the whole story. Menopause can grab us and tear us open in ways we couldn't have imagined before. The hot flashes and hot emotions seem to burn through a layer of "nice girl." You can find yourself more honest about who you really are, more fully yourself. Even if you do not change the shape of your outer life, your inner life *will* change.

A period of disorganization always precedes fundamental reorganization, and in both adolescence and menopause, this disorganization *begins with the body*. The body is the vessel, the crucible, for transforming who you are and preparing you for the next stage of your life. This should make a new kind of sense to you, given what I've said about how internal body changes transform your sense of self. Author Sarah Manguso, musing recently on the physiological nature of menopausal anger, asked, "What if, as menopausal women discover more forcefully than the rest of us, the duality of body and mind is simply irrelevant?"[31]

If you have been through menopause, perhaps you are now musing on your own passage. Maybe you're one of those people for whom menopause was particularly disruptive, and you were laid low by night (and day) sweats, mega-periods, and other physiological symptoms. Or you're someone for whom sexual attractiveness has been central to your identity, and you now feel like you've lost not only your sex appeal but also your power and even your value. Or perhaps you had fertility problems and had to go through a grueling series of reproductive technologies and now have to face the painful reality that your chance to have a biological child is truly over. And maybe . . . even if menopause was disruptive or distressing in certain ways, it was (or will be) also the time of your greatest awakening. It will help so much if you can truly take in the lessons and gifts of menopause and move into older age *consciously* with a mind open to surprises and new beginnings.

Older Age

Your body moves even closer to center stage some years later as you enter your seventies and eighties, and your body sense and body image are challenged once again. Aging can seem to come upon us suddenly, even though the process is gradual and slow. Our bones and muscles become less strong, affecting our balance and coordination. Our brain size gradually decreases, particularly in those parts of the brain responsible for short-term memory, processing speed, attentional focus, multitasking, hearing, and interoception. The diversity and resilience of the trillions of microbes in our gut decreases, making us a bit more vulnerable to various disorders, including, for some, Alzheimer's disease. While these changes are all part of the normal aging process, they must spur us to take excellent care of our older bodies, which I describe more throughout the book.

As we begin to experience these unwelcome changes in flesh, gut, joints, sensation, energy, thinking, and memory, we find ourselves struggling not only with feelings of loss or fear of encroaching mortality but also with a kind of dissonance between how we want to think of our bodies and how they actually appear and function. As one of my interviewees said, "I actually feel fine at this age as long as I don't have to look at myself in a mirror!" It will help us tremendously if we are able to respond to these new and disconcerting changes of aging with acceptance, even with tenderness and love.

It is also terribly important to notice and enjoy the many, many positive changes of aging, which I explore in chapter 7. We continue the transformations of self that began in menopause, becoming increasingly assertive and grounded, shaping our lives more around our own needs and fancies rather than those of others. And certain aging brain changes, which I'll discuss further later, actually lead to a mellowing of our emotions—a shift toward more positive emotional states and thus to a sense of greater well-being. We become happier and more optimistic. At my sixtieth birthday party, I joyfully told the group of friends assembled, "I can finally do what I damn well please!" We can discover important parts of ourselves we never knew existed and can finally give the parts of ourselves we already love their due. I have been able to recognize how deliriously happy music makes me and to really go after it and make room for it. I'd sung in vocal ensembles throughout my life, but I had never before really grasped that music was *necessary* to my happiness.

We're as variable in how we respond to getting older as to adolescence, menopause, or anything else. Like Nora Ephron, who titled her book *I Feel Bad About My Neck*, there may be things about your body that you feel particularly bad about. For you, it may be your balance, your inner-upper arms, your tummy, or your so-called invisibility. You may be someone who says, "Okay, I'm aging. That's the way it is. Nothing I can do about it." Or perhaps you are trying to delay the aging process as long as possible through exercise, nutrition, meditation, and so on. Or you may be someone who is working hard to delay the *look* of aging through skillful makeup techniques or cosmetic procedures of various kinds. Illnesses like heart disease or stroke may run in your family, which makes the prospect of aging a bit scarier for you. Or you may already have illnesses or physical disabilities, which is making the aging process more complicated or frightening.

My own position is clear, and it's very hopeful. You *can* keep on "remaking" your physical body by taking good care of it through exercise, diet, meditation, and so forth, and you can keep on remaking your *sense* of your body to bring it into alignment with your actual, ever-changing older body via the very same "body-making" processes I have described in this chapter. Holding and touch, mirroring affirmation, imitation, and movement remain crucial in reshaping and rethinking our sense of our older body. We need embodied interactions with others to keep our somatic and emotional selves invigorated and evolving throughout our lives. Mounting research makes it clear that our older brains are still, albeit to a lesser extent, "plastic," that is, capable of being changed through experience and practice. You may have "inherited" certain unfortunate tendencies or behaviors, but by working with your body as well as your mind, you can continue to transform yourself in positive ways. You can go on writing and rewriting your *inside story* until the very end.

One of the most hopeful insights I've gained doing research and interviews for this book is that *older age can actually be the time when we finally become more embodied.* Despite the age-related declines in body and brain functioning, it is my observation and strong belief that we older women are actually *primed* to experience our bodies more deeply and pleasurably. Why? Because our bodies are quieter and slower. There is less dramatic action inside the theater of our bodies without the cyclical hormonal changes and greater body/brain reactivity of our younger years. We are less impelled to *act* on our negative emotions. And the fact that our body is more fragile and needs more care and protection gives us a new opportunity to pay more attention to our body and to treat it with more kindness. If we can learn to bring positive attention to our body, we will be able to sense and feel it more and to really *dwell* in our body. In this way, we are naturally and continuously remaking our body sense and forging a more respectful and loving relationship with our body.

A Self-Guided Exercise

Write a letter to your body ("Dear body . . ."), reflecting upon how you have felt about your body from your earliest memories up to the present. Ask yourself some of the following questions, but don't feel limited by them:

- How did you feel about your body as a child? In your family, in school, in gym class?

- Was there physical affection in your family? How much?

- How did your mother/father/brothers/sisters respond to your body? Did they want you to look a particular way?

- Did you experience any trauma to your body, such as injuries, surgeries, or abuse?

- How did you feel about your body as a teenager? How did you react to puberty and the onset of menstruation?

- How did you feel about your body as a young and middle-aged adult?

- How important has your physical attractiveness been to you, in your job, in your circle of friends?

- How have you felt about being a sexual person, as a teenager, or a young, middle-aged, and older woman?

- How do you feel about your body now? Your body's aging?

- How does your spouse/partner feel about your aging and, specifically, your aging body?

- What is your relationship like with your body? How do you take care of your body?

- Do you feel attractive now? Do you think others find you attractive now?

- Are there certain parts or aspects of your body that you think about or worry about more than others?

- How much control do you feel you have over the aging process?

- How much do you think about aging and death?

Be sure to take some time for deep reflection as you write this letter to your body. Then you may want to change positions and write a letter from your body-you back to your mind-you, describing how your body-you feels you've been treated throughout your life. You may want to write your letter now, later, or not at all. But if you do, it can be interesting to observe how your relationship with your body changes as you read the rest of this book.

Chapter 4

The Emotional Body

As I write, COVID-19 is creeping its way around the globe. I'm living with feelings now I've never felt before, feelings I can't really put into words. There's a sort of darkness and blurriness that wasn't here before—a darkness all around me and inside me and a kind of tingly tightness, down my spine and in my stomach. The threat is "out there" somewhere, but where exactly? Everywhere! There's no safe place. What will happen to me, my family, my friends? What may already be happening to my body? What could happen to my husband, whose immune function is already compromised by a drug he's taking to control allergies? What could happen to my son, who's working in an industry considered "essential," so he can't shelter at home? I am frightened. What, exactly, should I be doing? There's an exhausting alertness, a need to stay aware of possible contagion points, to know more medical information, to plan more and better, to help more people, to do something more . . . but what? I feel baffled. And there's the added wrinkle (no pun intended) that I'm well over sixty and so am in the most vulnerable age group. That mean little virus is coming after us in particular. It's stalking us. In us it finds a welcoming host, a tasty treat. It's not fair. And yet . . . of course, we are always the most vulnerable. The frail old wildebeest falls in the savannah, left behind by the herd to get picked off by the hyenas. First to go, as it should be, always has been, always will be. We live closer to the truth of our mortality these days, closer to our humanity. COVID-19 is a slap across the face to take extra special care of this precious older body of mine. I must make my body as strong as possible and do as much as I can while I can. Carpe diem! I must guard this body with my life.

There is clearly a lot going on in my body and mind. My brain is registering my body sensations (darkness, blurriness, tingly tightness, alertness), and these sensations are triggering emotions (frightened, baffled) to help me try to make sense of which feelings are the most important ones to act on. My brain and my body are in constant, intense communication, one triggering the other. My feelings, they go round and round, while the painted ponies go up and down, and all of this, as I will now explain in more detail, is in the service of my continuing survival.

Emotions for Survival

All feelings are physical. Sensory signals from deep within your visceral body are continuously being received, integrated, encoded, and interpreted by your brain through the process I've already identified as *interoception*. It is this process of interoception, the sensing of ourselves from within, that determines our moods and mental states and general sense of well-being. As mentioned, neuroanatomists, starting with Bud Craig, have mapped in detail the neuroanatomical *interoceptive pathways*, which are akin to the pathways of our usual five external senses. They start with sensory receptors for touch, pressure, itch, temperature, and pain that are embedded in our internal organs, skin, hormonal system, digestive system, and immune system. They then progress through the vagus nerve to the top of the spinal cord, up through several locations in the upper brainstem and hypothalamus, where the interoceptive signals are processed and mapped to some degree, then up into the sensory-motor cortex at the very top of our brain to an area called the *insula*, where they are integrated and mapped in finer detail.[1]

These "supermaps" of your body sensations give you a sense of the physiological condition of your entire body, which you experience as your "emotions" and your sense of "self." Descartes's dictum was wrong. It's not "I think, therefore I am." What's true is "I *feel*, therefore I am." Your sense of being "you" comes from your body feelings! The new science of interoception, which has burgeoned over the past decade or two, provides confirmation of what our hallowed first psychologist, William James, first proposed in the 1860s, which later became known as the James-Lange theory: that our feelings are derived from sensing our body states. It also validates what Freud suggested in 1923: that the first "ego" is a body ego derived from body sensations. In our recent era, it is neuroscientist and philosopher Antonio Damasio who has definitively rooted human consciousness in the body.[2]

To reiterate, the fundamental purpose of gathering all this information from around the body is nothing less than the survival of the human organism. The brain is constantly monitoring your inner and outer worlds to help you maintain your physiological equilibrium, or *homeostasis*, and keep you alive and well. Your brain tries to figure out what all your inner sensations mean, based on information it receives from the *outside* world through your five senses and also based on memories of past experience stored in your brain. From all this it creates *emotions*, like anger, joy, sadness, disgust. Our emotions are not responses to objective situations but to what we *think* is happening.

Changes in your body state are picked up through your interoceptive pathways and recorded and mapped in important sites in your brainstem, like the periacqueductal gray, and in your cortex, particularly the anterior cingulate cortex, and the anterior insula. If these changes are cause for alarm, they trigger corrective physiological responses. Having a "felt experience" of the positive or negative quality of your bodily state allows you to quickly detect and correct any potentially dangerous physiological changes, like blood sugar imbalance. It also allows you to *predict* future adverse or favorable conditions. In other words, the main reason feelings and emotions emerged in our human evolution was to help us maintain our body's healthy equilibrium. *This* is why we have feelings.

As mentioned, our minds have a particularly powerful emotional connection with our guts, including the trillions of microorganisms that reside there. Emeran Mayer,[3] gastroenterologist and pioneer in the expanding new field of brain-gut microbiome research, explains that our gut is our largest sensory organ, with its own nervous system (the "enteric nervous system"). It remains in continuous biochemical dialogue with our brain, mainly through the vagus nerve. We've all experienced the connection between our mind and our gut, of course, when we get butterflies in our stomach (even diarrhea) before giving a big presentation, or we get a "gut feeling" that someone we meet isn't trustworthy. But it's only been in the past decade that the new field of "microbiome research" has begun to revolutionize our understanding of how human *emotions* are created. The enteric nervous system is now recognized as our "second brain" because it operates independently to regulate intestinal movement and analyze the food we ingest and figure out how to optimally digest it or reject it. But what is most surprising is that our gut, along with its trillions of microbes, is also constantly affecting our emotional well-being—even our social behavior, decision making, and perceptions of the world around us! When the communication system between brain, gut, and microbiome is disordered, major health problems can ensue, including not only digestive and autoimmune disorders like irritable bowel syndrome, but also anxiety and depression. The body is a vast symbiotic ecosystem of organisms, like the rain forest. When that ecosystem is disrupted by, say, antibiotics, there can be serious consequences.

It is humbling to note that our much-vaunted cerebral cortex contributes to but is not *essential* for the emergence of feelings, since feelings are activated in our body, even in our "lowly" gut, and first emerge in more "primitive" regions of the brain, like the brainstem. This means that feelings are not exclusive to humans or even mammals and may even be shared by birds and some reptiles.

Indeed, our body seems to be *more* savvy when it comes to picking up *patterns* of emotional experience, patterns that are too multifaceted to be held in our conscious minds. So, for example, when we revisit our elementary school after many, many years, we get "that feeling" in our bodies—maybe, a tightening in the abdomen, a shiver up the spine or across the back—that tells us something about what that period of our life was like for us. Our body remembers before we do, and it remembers more than we do. We cannot put "that feeling" about our elementary school into words or even thoughts, because there's just too much to be held in our conscious minds. "That feeling" remains in the body yet communicates multitudes about who we were at that point in our lives.

Emotions Versus Feelings

How is an emotion different from a feeling? A *feeling* is a sensation we experience as coming from our bodies—like my feeling of tingly tightness at the beginning of the COVID-19 pandemic. An *emotion*, grounded in our bodily sensations, also contains an *evaluation* of those feelings (how good or bad something feels to us) and is accompanied by some *urge to act*. The orbitofrontal cortex, a part of the frontal cortex located just above our eyes, is a major player in appraising our body states and what actions to take. And the orbitofrontal cortex teams up with the anterior cingulate cortex to generate a *motor* response, by harnessing our emotions to motivate us to take action.

> As I lie on my mat, Karen, my yoga instructor, takes me on a journey through my body, asking me to experience the sensations in every part of me. I feel the ache in that ankle I sprained four months ago, which tells me that playing tennis yesterday was not a wise idea and that I need to go easy on that ankle for a good while longer. I feel a tightness in my gut, which tells me that something may be out of whack with all those little beasties in my microbiome and that I need to relax more and eat more probiotic foods like yogurt or miso soup. Then, when we get to my neck, I can feel tension and pain, which informs me that I've been spending too much time writing at the computer and that I need to adjust my chair and posture and take more breaks to stretch and shake out my body.

My body sensations are telling me what's going wrong in my body and how to correct my behavior to make myself feel better and preserve my body. This process is going on all the time outside of my awareness, but, with my yoga instructor's help, I'm getting better and better at bringing it into my awareness.

"The advent of feelings was simultaneously the advent of the mind," Damasio writes. "Early organisms capable of feeling were for the first time in evolution aware of some aspect of their own existence. Feelings paved the way for the establishment of higher levels of cognition and consciousness, culminating in the modern human mind."[4]

How Emotions Are Created

The discovery of *simulation* during the 1990s has added another piece to the puzzle of how our emotions are created. Our brains are constantly creating *simulations* or imaginings or "guesses" about our environment and then making predictions about what will happen. For example, if I mention the words apple pie—voila!—there it is before you in all its plump, crusty glory, and if you're really hungry, you may even sense its delightful smell and taste. Your brain is basically a "prediction machine," according to neuroscientist Anil Seth.[5] It is constantly producing predictions and simulations, like video clips, of the outside world, derived from *concepts*, like emotions. *Emotions*, based on past experiences, are some of the most important concepts that give meaning to your experiences/sensations. Your brain compares your "video clip," your prediction, with the real-world situation coming in via sensory input. If there is a mismatch, what's called a "prediction error," you either have to change the concept or reevaluate or change the sensory input from your environment. By constantly predicting and simulating and correcting, we create our own world.

Here's an example. Let's say you're walking down a dark, unfamiliar street at night, when you hear footsteps behind you. Based on past experience (or movies), your brain predicts and simulates an attacker and starts to prepare your body for action. Your heart rate increases, you start to breathe more deeply, and you begin to feel shaky. You interpret all these physiological changes as "fear." But then let's say the footsteps slow slightly and begin to move away from you. You turn and see an older woman in a tan raincoat go into a doorway. Whew! Your brain corrects its faulty prediction, and your body calms down. In fact, your brain is continually producing predictions and simulations, which are attempts to "explain" our sensations/experiences through "concepts" like emotions (fear, in the above example). And these emotions, like disgust, fear, anger, sadness, joy, shame, contempt, pride, compassion, and admiration, are mostly triggered by the perception or recall of *exteroceptive* stimuli, like the sound of footsteps behind you on a dark street. Your brain uses this very same simulation process to make meaning of the sensations from *inside* your body, like your heartbeat or your breathing. Let's say you're waiting at the airport to greet your daughter, who's returning after three years abroad, and you notice that you're short of breath. You'll probably assume that it's because of your *excitement* about seeing your daughter. However, if you're "sheltering in place" during 2020–2021, you might well experience your shortness of breath as a sign that you've contracted COVID-19 and will experience *fear*. Your brain is using an *emotion concept*, based on your experience, to give meaning to your shortness of breath. We create our own emotional experiences based on internal and external input and past experience. There's a continuous conversation between body sensations, mental predictions, and meaning making.

In short, your brain actively *constructs* emotion and prescribes action. Emotions are not reactions to the world: you *create* them, based on your own storehouse of unique and personal experiences. They emerge from the particularities of your unique body and brain wiring and experience of your environment, culture, and upbringing. This is why different people have different emotional responses to the same thing—for example, why some people reacted to directives from the government to "shelter in place" during the pandemic as protective, while others viewed it as an infringement on their basic right to freedom. In every moment of your life, your brain uses experience, organized as "concepts" or "categories," to guide your actions and give your sensations meaning—sometimes by creating instances of emotion.

It makes me think of how Tibetan Buddhists think of the world as a dream, "illusion," or "maya." At a workshop on "dream yoga" decades ago at the Nyingma Institute in Berkeley, I was encouraged to cultivate lucid dreaming, the process of being aware that you are dreaming. If you deeply grasp that you can transform your dreams, the Tibetans believe, you can better understand how you can change your emotional reality in waking life.

Neuroscience is also offering up a new view of *where* emotions are located in the brain. Until recently, we believed that there were different, distinct circuits hardwired into our brain for the five major emotions—joy, sadness, fear, anger, and disgust (some experts add a sixth, surprise)—which had distinct facial expressions that could be captured in standard photographs of each. It was as if there were five different personifications of the major emotions residing in the mind—just like in the mind of the girl named Riley in the Pixar/Disney 2015 movie *Inside Out*. Each of Riley's emotions have their own dramatic characters—Joy, Disgust, Sadness, Anger, and Fear—who struggle to help Riley get through the emotional chaos of her family's big move from the Midwest to San Francisco.[6] Well, it turns out that it's not that simple. Hundreds of brain-imaging studies of emotion from past decades show that emotions do not have particular "fingerprints" in the brain. What's true is that many different networks, at many different levels of the brain, are all working together to create our emotions. Neuroscientist Jaak Panksepp revolutionized our understanding of how emotions are created when he identified seven such "affective systems," for example, the "seeing system." These systems are the source of our basic emotional feelings as well as our deepest values and are remarkably similar across all mammalian species.[7]

Your brain is always searching for explanations for what's going on in your body, but, then again, sometimes body sensations are simply body sensations. For example, you may wake up feeling shaky and dismally low-energy and imagine you're falling into an emotional funk, when in reality you may be exhausted, dehydrated, or getting the flu. And if you imagine that you're depressed, you can also "feel" worse in your body, and on and on, looping in a closed system that makes you feel even worse. So, there are times when you have to purposely engage your thinking brain to determine whether you might be *mis*interpreting your body sensations and creating unnecessary angst; you may then be able to try on a different interpretation and dial down your emotions. "You're not at the mercy of mythical emotional circuits buried deep inside some ancient part of your brain," says emotion scientist Lisa Feldman Barrett. "You have a lot more control over your emotions than you think you do."[8]

Our Emotional Inheritance

I must also stress again that our emotions develop and continue to unfold and change in *relationship*. From the very beginning as infants, our somatic sensations emerge and are processed within us—but certainly not in isolation. Rather, they arise along with the sensations created by our caretakers as they hold, move, stroke, rock, and feed us. In fact, as mentioned, the infant experiences many of her caretakers' nurturing actions as arising in her *own* body, as if they were her *own* actions, before they gradually become represented mentally as part of her own "self."[9]

Our caretakers' ongoing responses to our early feeling states—their "interpreting" and naming of our feelings—help us create emotional concepts in our own minds. These feelings can then begin to come online as emotions: anger around six months; fear around ten months; defiance, joy, pride, and shame near the end of the second year; and guilt not until three years. Over time, as our emotions continue to be empathically understood and responded to accurately enough by our caretakers, we become more able to think about, verbally articulate, and differentiate our emotions from one another and, if all goes well enough in development, to integrate all of our emotional states into our sense of "me." However, when our emotional states are not recognized and accepted by our caretakers—as Riley's sadness was too upsetting to be tolerated by her family in *InsideOut*—then these emotions will be split off from our conscious awareness, and we'll have trouble acknowledging and handling these particular feelings for the rest of our lives.

Managing Our Emotions

Emotions, which are bodily experiences, are not themselves inherently positive or negative. It's your relationship to them, what you *do* with them, that makes them helpful or destructive. If you choose to blast someone to smithereens with your anger, it can obviously be devastating for that person. If you use your anger to stop a child from running into the street, it can be lifesaving.

At this point, most Western and Eastern emotion researchers agree that we can *learn* to better manage our emotions. How? Both schools are convinced that it's best to try to *accept* our emotions as much as we can. If we are scared, for example, it is not helpful to either deny that emotion ("I'm not scared") or to blindly act on it ("I'm scared! I've got to run away from this situation"). We do best if we acknowledge our fear, feel it fully, then engage our thinking brain to help determine whether we should act on our fear or reconsider it and alter our emotional reaction.

The experience of emotional "well-being" is being studied more and more by Western researchers seeking to integrate emotional wisdom from Eastern contemplative traditions. It has been defined in countless ways—feeling good, healthy, comfortable, happy, contented, having purpose and meaning. The experience of well-being, to my mind, is more of an emotional state than an emotion per se. I would call it a full-body state—experienced throughout the body—as compared to, say, distinct emotions like love or gratitude that are felt more focally in the heart. Well-being, which is sometimes called "eudemonia," must be distinguished from hedonia, or "happiness." Hedonic happiness is still the overarching goal in our culture. It most often refers to sensory pleasures, like sex, food, alcohol, or fame. Paradoxically, of course, those people who strive to create moment-to-moment happiness are the least happy, because it is unattainable.

According to Buddhist traditions, healthy emotional states of well-being can be "cultivated" through ongoing *awareness* of our physical and mental states. Cognitive psychologists more often describe this process as learning "mind management," to "regulate" your emotional states and reactions. Mental health doesn't just happen; it's something you *do*. Unhealthy thoughts or beliefs, like those related to racism, are like viruses. If you leave them untreated, they can spread and cause grievous harm.[10]

On the other hand, certain positive and healthy emotions, like compassion, gratitude, altruism, kindness, and love, can be studied and trained. Dacher Keltner, a psychology professor at my doctoral alma mater, UC Berkeley, founded a research center called the Greater Good, which has been a major force in turning emotion research in the direction of understanding how healthy emotions elevate our sense of well-being.

Interestingly, Keltner has a particular focus on the capacity for *awe*, which he thinks is a defining feature of human beings. He defines awe as "the feeling of being in the presence of something vast that transcends your understanding of the world," and which opens up your mind to exploration, discovery, and connection.[11] Because our love of nature is motivated by awe, Keltner believes it is the emotion most likely to help us combat climate change. What's more, mounting research in positive psychology is showing how taking certain simple *actions* can almost miraculously change our sense of well-being, sometimes for significant periods of time. I'll discuss this more in chapter 7.

Measuring Your Interoceptive Awareness

Interoception is going on continuously inside all of us, both in and out of awareness, and is the source of our physical well-being, our emotional life, and our sense of self. Some of us, of course, are more sensitive to our body sensations than others. Are you, for example, someone who can feel actual hunger "pangs" when you need to eat? Are you someone who can sense strong feelings in the region of your heart, like love or compassion? Can you sense and feel your whole body? If so, you would be described as having higher *interoceptive awareness* (IA), and, as a result, you're likely to make more informed decisions. However, IA is not predestined or static. Evidence continues to mount that IA can be developed through learning to focus inward and through various practices, which I continue to elaborate throughout this book.

How on earth do scientists study something like interoceptive awareness when they readily admit that it's very difficult to collect objective evidence of interoception? Many different facets of IA have been measured, including the ability to attend to, accurately monitor, and discriminate among internal sensations, but, for years now, the primary method has been through a measure of interoceptive "accuracy" (IAcc) called the *heartbeat counting task*. You are asked to silently count your heartbeats for several different durations while your heartbeat is being recorded using a "pulse oximeter," that little electronic device that doctors clip on your finger to measure the oxygen in your blood and your heart rate. There's also a test whereby you listen to a series of beeps through headphones and report whether you think the beeps are in time with your own heartbeats or not. In either test situation, some people are much better than others in detecting their heartbeats. It all began with a pioneering study in the early 1990s, when Hugo Critchley and his team discovered that people who were best at sensing their heartbeats had much more activity in the insula and other major sites of interoceptive activity in the brain.[12] Since then the various heartbeat detection tests have come under scrutiny for not always measuring what they set out to measure, but they remain the most common laboratory measure of IA.

There is also a popular questionnaire, the Multidimensional Assessment of Interoceptive Awareness (MAIA) that provides a subjective measure of IA. Developed by psychologist Wolf Mehling, this questionnaire taps into how aware you are of body sensations and the connection between body sensations and emotional states, how well you regulate distress by attending to body sensations and actively listening to your body for insight, and whether you experience your body as safe and trustworthy. Sample statements from the second version of the MAIA (2018)[13] include:

- When I am tense, I notice where the tension is located in my body.
- I notice when I'm uncomfortable in my body.
- I distract myself from sensations of discomfort.
- I am able to consciously focus on my body as a whole.
- I notice how my body changes when I get angry.
- I can use my breath to reduce tension.
- I listen to my body to inform me about what to do.

It turns out that people with higher interoceptive awareness, as measured by the MAIA, are mentally healthier. They have better emotion regulation, greater ability to be present in the moment ("presence") and affect change ("agency"), more empathy for others, firmer self/other boundaries, and better decision making, to name only the main results found across studies. We'll look at these more in chapter 6. It is interesting, however, that people who *report* greater IA do not necessarily score higher on objective measures like heartbeat detection.

I must add that there appear to be some gender differences in interoceptive awareness, which have largely been ignored in the research. One of the few studies that deliberately set out to study gender differences, using the MAIA, found that young adult females tended to notice bodily sensations more often, better understand the relation between body sensation and emotional states, experience more distress when they have pain or discomfort, and generally feel less safe.[14] These findings are in keeping with neuropsychiatrist Louann Brizendine's observations in her popular book *The Female Brain*, in which she describes women's greater sensitivity and reactivity to bodily states and emotions, which stems from our having larger and more active insulas.[15]

Disorders of Interoceptive Awareness

Many disorders, like anorexia, bulimia, panic disorder, body dysmorphia, post-traumatic stress disorder (PTSD), depression, drug addiction, psychosis, and perhaps even autism, can now be thought of as pathologies of interoceptive awareness. People with panic or anxiety disorders, for example, tend to have heightened interoceptive awareness, while people with PTSD are likely to have reduced IA. Many patients with PTSD have learned to shut off their visceral sensations, because they fear the welling up of overwhelming feelings like terror, despair, or acute physical pain. They are saying, in effect, *I can't afford to pay attention to what's there, because I have no control over it, and I can't expect to get any help with it.* People suffering in these ways use various strategies to *not* feel their bodies or to only feel their external bodies in a coercive way. All routinely recruit the psychological defense called dissociation to "numb out" or "space out" traumatic feelings, thoughts, or sensations.

Many individuals also use self-harm behaviors, like starving, binging, purging, substance abuse, self-cutting, or skin picking, to try to manage intolerable emotional pain. Paradoxically, many use self-harm behaviors not only to "not feel" but to feel *something in their bodies*. For example, my patient who delicately (not with suicidal intent) cut her inner arms with a razor blade could feel the sharp pain as relief, an intense alternative focus or distraction from overwhelming emotional distress. And because the acute pain can cut through the dissociative fog, it could temporarily make her feel more "real" and "alive."

With patients like these, who can no longer feel their bodies, I need to *actively* encourage them to develop their bodily awareness by asking them to notice what's happening in their bodies, both in the therapy session and outside. All of us, of course, can benefit tremendously from increasing our awareness of our body sensations—particularly since we now know that our body awareness is inextricably linked to our *emotional* awareness, our embodiment and sense of self. Interoceptive awareness is also linked to what is called "emotion tolerance," which is the ability to sit with your emotions without alarm or judgment or having to avoid, numb, or deny them. You can recognize and accept your feelings as important information, self-signals of changes in the state of your body/mind.

My patient Jenny, age fifty-two, was quite "deaf" to her body's sensations or communications and at different times had used an eating disorder or sedating medications to numb out her considerable anxiety. She had recently started a new job, which involved meetings all day over Zoom and writing a lot of reports online. She was a self-described "technophobe." As the days went by, she became more and more anxious and overwrought, saying, "I don't know what I'm doing. I don't know what to do." She began to work longer and longer hours, spending hours doing Zoom tutorials and writing and rewriting reports until she was too exhausted to concentrate but too revved up to relax. Jenny found herself doing the same things over and over without making progress, mired in fearful rumination about losing her mind and getting fired, as her gears continued to grind and slow. Her body was saying "no more" and shutting down, but her overtaxed mind just kept on trying to triumph over her bone-tired body.

There is only one way out of this awful state of neurophysiological depletion and emotional overwhelm, and that is *through the body*. Bottom-up. I suggested to Jenny that she immediately take a day off, drop everything, and begin radical self-care. I encouraged her to slow down her breathing and her movements and listen carefully to her body to determine when she needed to rest, work, move, stretch, eat. She discovered that long, slow, meandering walks, while looking deeply at the quiet beauty of the world around her, were amazingly restorative. When she finally began to slow down, she could reenter her body and feel its crushing exhaustion. Then she could finally begin to relax and sleep and heal.

Empathic Communication

We are continually responding viscerally to the emotions of others. Imagine you are listening to your old college chum speaking at her father's funeral. You hear her voice catch, then become husky, and suddenly you feel seized by your own distress. Or you see a look of disgust on someone's face as they sample a food, and you yourself feel a yucky sensation. In short, when you see joy, you can feel joy. When you see sadness, you can feel sadness. If you witness someone getting a shot in the arm, you actually feel the pain.

How do we explain this? How does one body "communicate" with another? Some of it can very simply be explained by what's commonly called "nonverbal communication"—"reading" the body language of others, picking up clues about their inner feelings from observing their body tension, restriction of breathing, tone of voice, and so on. To understand body-to-body communication more deeply, however, we must turn to that still-mysterious set of processes called *empathy*, the ability to experience the feelings of others.

In fact, there is now a "neuroscience of empathy," much of which focuses on physical or emotional pain. This research, using fMRI brain scans, consistently shows that when you view the suffering of other people, you activate the same neural circuit as when you experience your own emotional distress.[16] So, seeing the suffering of others really does cause you to suffer as well. When you observe other people in physical pain, however, only the affective (emotional) networks for pain are activated, not the sensory ones, so you don't literally feel their pain. This "empathy circuit" in your brain cortex includes the insula and the anterior cingulate, which, you recall, process sensory information from all over your body, so it follows that raising your interoceptive awareness makes you better at empathizing. Having a template for a feeling in your own body allows you to more easily predict and simulate a feeling in another person's body.

How do we develop this ability to empathize? I have described how when we are infants, the "affective touch" of our mothers and other primary caretakers allows us to experience our mother's body as part of our own, her interoceptive abilities as our own. As you grow up and differentiate yourself from others, you still retain the ability to have momentary experiences of self-other fusion—particularly, studies show, when our bodily movements and sensations are in *synchrony* with those of another. You can see the synchrony in the brain scans: there is activation in both *your* insula and in that of the other. But empathy requires more than these temporary feelings of fusion. You must be separate enough to be able to determine the *origin* of a given feeling—in other words, where (in *whom*) the feeling originated. Not having a clear sense of the origin of emotions can make us too "porous" and vulnerable to "emotional contagion" and is related to low interoceptive awareness.[17]

And what about those *mirror neurons* sprinkled throughout your brain, which are involved in your being able to "mirror" others' behavior in your own brain? A mirror neuron, you'll recall from chapter 3, is a neuron that automatically fires both when you perform an action and when you *see someone else* perform the same action. Remember the macaque monkey in Giacomo Rizzolatti's lab watching a scientist eat a peanut and having the same "peanut-eating" neurons fire in his *own* motor cortex? Soon after this revolutionary discovery in the early 1990s, scientists and journalists began exploring mirror neurons as the source of imitation—especially imitative learning in children—and, in addition, they hailed mirror neurons as the source of human empathy and attunement.[18] But now, three decades and dozens of studies later, scientists still have not found consistent evidence that what is now called the "mirror system" in humans is the source of empathy. They have, however, made an interesting distinction between two different forms of empathy: (1) the affective/perceptual type—sensing or feeling what someone else is feeling; and (2) the cognitive-evaluative type—*knowing* what someone else is thinking or feeling, even if you don't sense it yourself. The mirror system is more involved in the second, cognitive/evaluative type of empathy.[19]

Body-to-Body Communication

In my own field of relational psychoanalysis, we have at long last become aware that there are two *bodies* as well as two minds in the consulting room. Many of us now believe that the "unconscious" is not, as Freud believed, a part of the mind that houses forbidden or other repressed thoughts but is, instead, a register of the mind that is often not conscious because it is *bodily*.[20] The renegade Hungarian psychoanalyst Sandor Ferenczi was the first to pay close attention to the body-to-body communication that is always taking place between therapist and patient. As psychotherapists, we are now trained to consciously and deliberately attend to our *own* body sensations, as well as lots of other information, to get a sense of what feelings our patients may be holding in their bodies, like in a constricted gut, but not in their conscious minds, so we can help them retrieve and process those experiences. Over years and years of doing psychotherapy, my bodily self has become much more adept at sensing my patients' warded-off emotional states.

Each time my patient Tiffany, now fifty-seven, begins to move into an unspeakably traumatic adolescent memory of being drugged, sexually assaulted, and abandoned in a threatening and unfamiliar neighborhood, I find myself plunging into a very particular, intense bodily state. As she describes in a tiny and halting voice what she went through on that awful night, I feel frozen and paralyzed, yet utterly heartbroken. I feel afraid to breathe. I feel unbearable sadness and heaviness in my body. I find myself leaning far forward in my chair, trying somehow to magically envelope her body with my body to comfort and protect her.

I think of another patient, Christine, age forty-nine, who, like Tiffany, has very little internal body awareness. As a child, she had to endure frequent and terrifying emotional abuse by her psychotic mother. As an adult, she has dramatic mood swings, and, when most upset, she will often binge for hours at a time on low-calorie vegetable snacks. When I tried to explore her eating disorder, Christine would become enraged, because, as her primary survival strategy, it had to be defended at all costs. At one point, when I was feeling a bit hopeless about making progress with her treatment, something very interesting began to change in the way she described her binging behavior. At first, she said, "I eat and eat and eat," then she began saying, "I eat and eat and eat and eat and eat," then, finally, "I eat and eat and eat and eat and eat and eat and eat and eat and eat." Each iteration would grind into my abdomen. What was Christine trying to tell me? Finally, I wondered if she was trying to give me *her* experience of being forcibly stuffed with food, and she said, "Yes! Maybe. . . . It feels *awful*."

Christine had grabbed hold of me with her incessant repetitions and made me feel in *my* body the awful relentlessness of her stuffing *her* body. On a more profound level, she communicated something about how her mind felt as a child as it was oppressively stuffed with crazy, destructive, ideas by her mother. Looked at in retrospect, that moment could be seen as a turning point. My shifting my focus to what I was aware of in *my* body seemed to get Christine more in touch with what was going on inside *her* body and mind.

We Get More Positive with Age

A fascinating paradox arises as we get older. While we all, to lesser or greater degrees, lose some of our cognitive sharpness, we do, at the same time, get more adept at regulating our *emotions*, particularly our negative ones. "In terms of emotion, the best years come late in life,"[21] declares Laura Carstensen, founding director of the Stanford Center on Longevity, who has spent the past thirty years investigating the psychology of aging. She loves to debunk what she calls "the misery myth" that older people are sad, lonely, and dejected, and she points out that with the exception of dementia-related cases, mental health generally *improves* with age. We older people as a group suffer less from depression, anxiety, and substance abuse and have fewer negative emotions. When we do have negative emotions, we manage them better than younger people do. We are also able to experience more mixed emotions—for example, sadness and happiness at the same time. We're more comfortable with feelings of sadness and anger, and we're better at dealing with hotly charged emotional conflicts and debates. We direct our attention and memory to positive information more than negative. If you show people of all ages positive and negative images and ask them to recall all the images they can, older people remember more positive than negative images Carstensen calls this the "positivity bias." And it's the most cognitively sharp older adults who show this positivity effect the most.

(I wonder if this "positivity bias" of older age is in some part a result of a decrease in the well-known "negativity bias," which refers to our universal human proclivity to attend to, remember, and learn more from negative information, like insults, injuries, or traumatic events. The negativity bias is thought to serve an adaptive evolutionary function by keeping us on the lookout for threats to our survival, but perhaps, as we age, natural selection is less interested in our continuing survival!)

At one point in her research career, Carstensen wondered if maybe our older generation was just unusually positive. Perhaps the young people of today might not feel more positive as they got older. In a remarkably ambitious study, she and colleagues followed the same group of people, ages eighteen to ninety-four at the beginning of the study, over a ten-year period to see whether their emotional experience would change as they grew older. Each participant carried a beeper, and the investigators would page them throughout the day and evening at random times, asking questions like: "On a 1 to 7 point scale, how happy are you right now?" "How sad are you right now?" "How frustrated are you right now?" And what she and her colleagues learned was that, yes, the same individuals over time *do* report relatively greater positive experiences as they get older. Another important study widened the time window even more and was able to show that emotional stability gradually improved over *seven decades* (ages twelve to seventy-nine) of the human life span.[22]

Why Do We Mellow?

Why do older people feel more positive than people in the "prime of their lives"? Many have asked this question. Carstensen's explanation has to do with perspective. Recognizing that we don't live forever changes our perspective on life, and we are increasingly motivated to savor the time that is left by focusing on that which is emotionally meaningful. Her theory, called "socioemotional selectivity theory," has been widely confirmed.

Other researchers, however, have offered alternative (or additional) explanations for Carstensen's findings that aging brings greater well-being. One influential team of researchers[23] proposed in their Aging Brain Model that age-related changes in brain function can explain why older people view the world more positively. The main actor is the amygdala, the brain region most involved in emotion. The amygdala declines with age and becomes less reactive to negative stimuli, thereby elevating our sense of well-being. (Amygdala activation to positive stimuli stays the same across age.) A competing line of neuroscientific research posits that older people tend to be more positive because we are able to take more cognitive, higher-brain control of our emotions, to change our focus of attention and direct it toward more positive goals or memories. Brain scans do confirm that the two areas associated with selective attention and cognitive control (the ventral medial prefrontal cortex and adjacent anterior cingulate cortex) are more active in older adults than younger ones.[24] It may well be that all three explanations are true and working in tandem: that is, a less reactive amygdala, along with a shift toward taking more cognitive control of negative stimuli, plus an altered time perspective allow us to have a better regulated, more positive emotional life and a greater sense of well-being. And there is another factor.

Aging and Body Sense

It will not surprise you to learn that our *interoceptive awareness* also declines with age, as sensory signals throughout our body get weaker.[25] This muting of our internal bodily sensations comes with many downsides, of course, like hearing or vision loss, but it also has a significant upside when it comes to our sense of well-being. Our *emotions* become less activating. Several striking recent studies show that older people's emotional experience is not as linked to internal body signals as it is in younger adults—particularly for high-arousal emotions like anger and fear.[26] In experiments designed to trigger high-arousal emotions like anger or fear, we older folks are much less likely to experience intense sensations like "heart racing" or "blood pumping" than younger people.[27] Does this jibe with your experience? It does with mine. I can still remember my pounding heart and clammy hands before exams in college. What a relief to have a less reactive body!

And yet . . . how does this square with the many findings that *higher* interoceptive awareness is linked to so many measures of well-being—or, for that matter, with my own experience that my body awareness has *increased* as I've gotten older? I asked Sahib Khalsa, the psychiatrist and neurophysiologist whose 2009 study proved that interoception declines with age, and here's what he said: "Look, Susan, you wear glasses, right? You know you can't change the shape of your eyeball or lens without surgery, so, in the same way, you can't change that basic sensory signal which attenuates with age. But you can change how you *perceive* it. You can change what you *do* with it."[28]

Khalsa referenced Walter Cannon, the great physiologist of the 1930s, who believed that one of the unique characteristics of aging is wisdom. "What he may have meant by wisdom," Khalsa told me, "is that you learn through experience over time how to more effectively navigate your physical and emotional environments. Over the course of five, six, seven, eight, nine decades, you learn how to more quickly connect a body sensation with your subsequent feeling—for example, 'Oh dear, I know that every time I have to go meet with that person, I get this yucky feeling in my body, so I'm going to reflect on that and adopt a different strategy.' With wisdom, you have an integrated set of representations about your body to draw upon in evaluating your sensations and deciding what to do with your feelings."

What this means is that although your basic body sensations are not as strong as you age, your "wisdom" allows you to interpret them better. We can better recognize, understand, and manage our emotions and those of others. This is undoubtedly one reason why so many cultures across time, less youth-obsessed and speedy than ours, have looked to their elders for calming and guidance. We'll look more at what you can *do* with your inner sensations in chapter 5, when I discuss how to build body awareness.

As I was writing about how older people are more able to let go of life's negatives and focus on the positives, my friend Susan wrote to cancel our book group due to the rapidly spreading pandemic. She ended her email with, "In the meantime, I think we all need some Nina Simone!" and appended a link to Simone's song "Ain't Got No, I Got Life," in which the singer rattles off all the things she "ain't got" in her down-and-out life, but then joyfully enumerates two dozen parts of her body that she "got" and concludes with a triumphant "I got my freedom" and "I got life!" Listen to Nina Simone now on your favorite platform—we do need her!

As we all know, aging is not a walk in the park. For everyone, there is change, gradual loss, and, over time, sometimes tremendous loss. For many, there is disability, and for some, loneliness and depression. This is particularly true when our body starts to give us some trouble, and we fall into a particular emotional bog that is, unfortunately, all too common: we confuse physical problems, even minor issues, like aches upon awakening, with aging. A good example is my sixty-eight-year-old interviewee Julie. When I asked her how she feels about getting older, she said:

> Humbling is the word. It depends on what's going on with my body. When I turned fifty-eight, I made a decision to start doing good stuff for my body, and I decided to go to a masseuse, but the masseuse did something terrible to my hip and I got bad sciatica. I was suddenly in a lot of pain, and it catalyzed this whole downward spiral. I got thrown into the deep end with no warning, and I got very depressed. I went to see a lot of doctors and was finally told I needed a hip replacement. I got it replaced . . . but I'm still in and out of pain. And when I have pain, I think, "Oh, I'm going to die."
>
> All this threw me into aging in a big way. I'm not comfortable any place. I decided to go on this cruise because I thought that would be a place where I could be comfortable. I was with all these older people, and we're watching this entertainment event, and here I am completely restless and moving all the time and they're all able to sit still. I still don't remember what it's like to be young. When we're with our friends who are in their seventies I feel like I'm more in their frame of mind.

So, here we see Julie, suddenly feeling "old" at fifty-eight because a masseuse injured her body! To this day, she is still confusing a very unfortunate intervention with the aging process. Julie is experiencing pain sensations from a bodily injury, which are being interpreted by her brain as "I'm old" and serving as emotional predictions that she is nearing the end of her life. What a boggy cycle! I will show you later in the book how to use your body awareness to address your aches and pains—and sometimes to fix them!

Chapter 5

Moving from Outside to Inside

Gina, age forty-nine, believed she could be seen as appealing, or even acceptable, only if she was extremely thin, had every hair in place, and had not a single wrinkle in her clothing. If she was having a "bad-hair day," she found it hard to think about anything else and hid from people in the outside world. If her abdomen was "sticking out," she was sure everyone, including me, was focusing only on that. She had drawn up and posted on her closet door lists of the attributes of the perfect social person, the perfect daughter, the perfect wife, and the perfect career person, each with its own particular clothing, shoes, hairstyle, and mannerisms. Without the lists, Gina told me, she did not know how to "be."

We've come to believe that no matter what's ailing us—whether we're worried, sad, low-energy, angry, unmotivated, feeling "old"—we can feel better if we change our *body* in some way. A new hair color? A new body weight (usually thinner)? Some fabulous new shoes, even though they kill my feet? Some Botox to get rid of that frown (which makes me look old)? And now that I think of it, why not a "mini-facelift"? Over the past couple of decades, omnipresent, globalized visual media, coupled with an "aging industrial complex," have buried us in images of an ideal, young, slender, Westernized woman, and we have fallen for it hook, line, and wrinkle-filler.

Actually, it started even earlier. You may remember that wildly successful Virginia Slims advertising campaign launched in 1968 by Philip Morris, specifically marketed to "liberated" women with the slogan "You've come a long way, baby!" The ads featured a very slim cigarette held by a very slim, sexy "new" woman in trendy designer clothes; in the background were unappealing images of repressed, traditional women from the past. The message was clear: you too can be a slim, sexy, "independent" woman (if you get jacked up enough on the nicotine in these cigarettes). Women were literally dying to be thin.

Our society clearly cares a lot more about how we women look than how we feel. Yes, there are small sectors of our society, like the yoga, Pilates, or meditation communities, that encourage us to go inward and pay attention to how we actually feel in our bodies. But our culture's hungry gaze is directed primarily toward our *outer* body, which other people see and evaluate—to the point that it's considered part of female gender identity to be preoccupied with our physical appearance and sexual attractiveness. Meanwhile, the $200 billion anti-aging industry keeps chugging along, conniving to sell anti-aging products by making all of us over forty feel insecure, ashamed, or even disgusted by our less taut and smooth bodies and faces.

We have to combat this insidious fixation on the young, perfected, female body and put *ourselves* in charge of how we understand, view, present, and experience our own bodies. We need to further the revolution started in 1970 with the publication of the now classic book *Our Bodies, Ourselves,*[1] which inspired women to take control of our own bodies, particularly our health care and sexuality. Now, a half-century later, we must take charge of our *aging* bodies and selves by honoring the acumen of our older somas, and by defining for ourselves how *we* want to look and feel in our older years.

Endless Remodeling

What's new and particularly insidious in today's culture is that the body is viewed as a crucial and ongoing personal "project," as Susie Orbach suggests in her book *Bodies.* Our bodies are to be honed, altered, transformed, and perfected through exercise, dieting, cosmetic surgery, injections, implants, peels, and, more recently, Photoshop. Our bodies are viewed as canvases upon which to paint the perfect, attractive image of ourselves. According to Orbach, our bodies have become a form of work. The body has become "an object, a site of production and commerce in and of itself. Instead of our bodies making things, we now make our bodies."[2]

Of course, we all want to look and feel attractive and healthy. What's notable about our modern society is that we want to look a particular *kind* of attractive: we want to pass for *younger* than we are. *We want to outrun time.* All this creates tremendous body insecurity and anxiety about aging and leaves us unable to settle into and actually "live in" the body we have right now. Plastic surgeons are now warning younger women and men that aging starts early, and they suggest beginning cosmetic surgery in our thirties. "Start early, do often" is the motto. In certain areas of the country, like Los Angeles, women are accused of "letting themselves go" if they don't remodel themselves constantly.

For a short time, I worked with a sixty-six-year-old patient, Maggie, who was very wealthy and addicted to plastic surgery, which she saw as "fun" and a "treat to myself." She had already had six separate surgical procedures on her face. She would often encourage me to try it, looking pityingly at my wrinkles and sags. The worst part of it for me was that she had had first-rate plastic surgery, so she looked really good, and I found myself feeling envy at times. What a contradiction! I maintain that I don't want to have plastic surgery but then feel envious when surgery makes my patient look "better"—that is, younger. With my friends, it's the same thing. They say, "Oh no, I don't want to have 'work' done," but then, invariably, they all make this identical little move, where they quickly push up the skin in front of both ears, lifting the sagging skin on jowl and neck. It makes me sigh. So many of us are in the grip of this thing.

It must be acknowledged that the body positivity movement has, in the past decade, taken some admirable strides toward its stated goal of promoting acceptance of bodies of all sizes and shapes—including full-size models in clothing ads, a "Curvy Barbie" doll, and fewer weight-based descriptions of women in the media—but we're certainly not there yet. The pressure for women to project a thin, vibrant, sexual image continues to proliferate with each new form of social media.

In fact, the ideal body size and reality are moving further and further apart. The weight of the most famous fashion models, whose images are omnipresent, and the weight of the average woman continue to diverge, according to studies of body mass index (BMI), a calculation of a person's amount of body fat (weight divided by height in kilograms). The most famous thinnest have gotten thinner. A recent survey[3] of ten top international fashion models shows they had an average BMI of 17, when the normal range for BMI is between 18.5 and 25. In fact, Kendall Jenner, Adriana Lima, and Alessandra Ambrosio had BMIs of 16, and Karlie Kloss, Miranda Kerr, Cara Delevingne, and Doutzen Kroes had BMIs of 17, which are classified by the World Health Organization as "seriously underweight" and implicated in osteoporosis and anemia, hair loss and muscle wasting, respiratory disease, and lowered immune function. At the very same time, the average weight of the average 5-foot-4-inch American woman has gone up to 170.6 pounds, with a BMI of 29.6, in the "overweight" range,[4] which can also have serious health consequences, like high blood pressure, high blood cholesterol, increased risk of diabetes, joint pain, and fatigue. Almost three-quarters of both female and male Americans are classified as overweight, giving North America the highest percentage of any continent worldwide.

Think about it. The average woman just keeps getting heavier for myriad sociocultural reasons, while top fashion models remain at the same sad low weight for the past several decades. Neither extreme is good for us.

Body Image and Well-Being

As discussed in chapter 3, *body image* refers to the imagined body—how we visualize and experience our external body in our mind's eye and how we imagine it in the eyes of others. According to body image expert Thomas Cash, body image has three components: (1) the perceptual, which is your estimation of your own body size and its accuracy relative to your actual proportions; (2) the affective dimension, which involves your positive or negative feelings toward your bodily appearance; and (3) your beliefs about body shape and appearance.[5] Each of these three dimensions appears to have a distinct neural network. Body image itself is two things:

an "online," moment-to-moment, changing mental representation of your body and a more stable, more general representation of the structure of your body. A positive body image is critically linked to well-being.

How women feel about their bodies is explored through scientific studies of body image—usually focused on what's termed "body dissatisfaction," which is defined as the negative thoughts and feelings you have about your body. It's hard to get an exact read on how many women experience body dissatisfaction, because the diversity of the many tests used to study it make comparisons difficult. But overall, we can estimate that somewhere between 69 percent and 84 percent of adult American women of all ages report being dissatisfied with their bodies. One of the largest studies of body image satisfaction over the entire adult life span,[6] involving six thousand women, found that the vast majority of women (almost 91 percent) have a preferred body size that is smaller than their current body size. Studies show that "midlife" women (ages 42–52) are particularly vulnerable to body dissatisfaction, most probably because the weight increase of middle age widens the discrepancy between the actual body and the "thin ideal." Midlife women who are dissatisfied with their bodies are *twice* as likely to report clinically significant depression symptoms.[7] It gets a bit better as we get older, which I'll say more about shortly, but sadly enough, a negative view of one's body must be considered "normative" for females in our current society.

Body Dissatisfaction Has Increased

It was not always thus. American women's satisfaction with their bodies only started seriously tanking around sixty years ago—especially from 1959 through 1979, when the ideal female body got precipitously thinner. Using body measurements of *Playboy* centerfold models and Miss America contestants, researchers documented that what they called "model women" (that is, models for other women) had become significantly thinner.[8] They also showed that a sharp increase in diet articles and in eating disorders could be directly linked to our culture's rising expectations for thinness. By the mid-1990s, the female beauty ideal had become synonymous with the "thin ideal," as it has remained ever since, despite abundant evidence that the "thin ideal" breeds body hatred, negative mood, constant dieting, and eating disorders.

> It is the year 2008 and Sarah Michelle Gellar, star of the "Buffy the Vampire Slayer" TV series, walks on stage to the wild screaming of some three hundred middle-school girls and their parents. We're at a conference in San Jose designed to improve body image and self-esteem, and I'm one of the parent trainers. Gellar reads a moving and excruciating segment from the diary of a twelve-year-old girl, describing her eating disorder and body hatred. "I am so ugly . . . I just want to hide." Then this beautiful and overwhelmingly popular young actress tells the audience that this was *her* diary. Gasps and exclamations rumble through the room, then dead silence. Gellar has powerfully made her point—that hardly any female escapes the scourge of body hatred in our culture.

There is also a new wrinkle. Sometime around 2010, media images began promoting bodies that were muscular and toned as well as thin—a trend some have dubbed "fitspiration," a takeoff on "thinspiration." To study this new trend, a research team presented sixty-four undergraduate women with images of thin, muscular bodies side-by-side with images of the same bodies with the muscularity digitally removed, and they found that the participants overwhelmingly preferred the more muscular bodies. Looking at these images of muscular-and-thin women also heightened the women's negative mood and lowered their body satisfaction. Lead researcher Frances Bozsik writes, "It seems to add another layer of pressure, another thing to strive for . . . because there's a deceitful aspect of rhetoric surrounding 'fitspiration,' with benign implications that it's simply all about being healthy. We fear that our culture may be in the midst of a more toxic promotion of an ideal female body that only leads to more dissatisfaction."[9]

Body dissatisfaction is a major risk factor for eating disorders, depression, low self-esteem, and even suicidal ideation among adolescents.[10] It is estimated that 9 percent, or 28.8 million Americans, two-thirds of them women, will have a diagnosable eating disorder sometime in their lifetime.[11] The percentages of eating disorders are highest among college students (with a range of 8–17 percent), followed by teens ages 15 to 17 (about 4 percent). Not surprisingly, elite female athletes are particularly at risk, with more than a third in the Division 1 NCAA having some attitudes and symptoms of anorexia.

Contrary to popular belief, diagnosable eating disorders do not only occur in teenage girls and young women but in women and men across the life span. Most interesting for us is the estimate that 13 percent of women older than fifty engage in disordered eating behaviors. In fact, I have seen dozens of them over the years in my psychotherapy practice. I must stress that these figures do not take into account "subclinical" (nondiagnosable) eating disorders, which manifest, for example, as constant weight concern, aberrant eating patterns, or misperception of one's weight. Sadly, subclinical eating disorders appear to occur in a preponderance of women of all ages and ethnicities.

One of the best-known body image questionnaire studies is the 1997 *Psychology Today* survey of four thousand people, of which 90 percent were women.[12] In this study, 56 percent of women said they were dissatisfied with their overall appearance. Which parts of their bodies did they like the least? Most (71 percent) said their abdomen, followed by their body weight (66 percent), hips (60 percent), and muscle tone (58 percent). Looking at their abdomens in the mirror was rated as the most depressing experience for 44 percent of women—compared to looking at their faces, for only 16 percent. When respondents were asked what made them feel better about their bodies, they said, "good sex" and "exercising just for the pleasure of it."

It is also notable that the overwhelming majority of all respondents—93 percent of women, 89 percent of men—said they want models in magazines to represent the natural range of body shapes . . . even though most still believe that clothes look better on thin models. If you're interested, take a look at the original questionnaire at psychologytoday.com.

Feminism and Body Image

Feminist theory would suggest that feminists are less likely to objectify themselves and evaluate their appearance by societal standards. So, you may ask, are women who identify themselves as feminists at all protected from our society's widespread body image problems? A well-designed study of 1,241 racially and ethnically diverse young women (ages twenty to thirty-one) looked at the relationship of feminist identity, body image concerns, and disordered eating.[13] The researchers found that the 14.5 percent of participants who self-identified as feminists did indeed report significantly higher body satisfaction than nonfeminist women (36 percent) or a third group of women who held feminist beliefs but did not *self-identify* as feminists (49.9 percent). In a meta-analysis of twenty-four other studies of feminism and body image, the most powerful finding was that feminists (particularly older ones) had the lowest ratings on body shame and internalization of the media image. The aforementioned *Psychology Today* study also found that participants who called themselves feminist (32 percent of the total) were much less likely to be strongly dissatisfied with their overall appearance than traditional women (49 percent). When asked more specifically about their *weight*, only 24 percent of feminists, compared to 40 percent of traditional women, were extremely dissatisfied. Moreover, traditional women were twice as likely to report vomiting to control their weight as women who described themselves as feminists.

Why are feminists more able to withstand the pervasive societal pressures of our sexist and image-conscious society? For one thing, feminist theory denounces gendered power relationships, so women who identify as feminists are more able to dismiss the unrealistic and unhealthy body ideals perpetrated by men and the male-dominated media.[14] I myself think more broadly in terms of *sense of self*. Those of us who ardently believe in and advocate for equal rights and opportunities for women feel more empowered to determine the shape of our own lives, including the image we present to the world. Whatever the reasons, these findings that feminists have more positive body images are extremely important, because they can encourage influential people in all corners of society—educators, parents, eating disorder therapists, public policy makers, politicians—to work harder to advance beliefs and practices that encourage women to define their *own* bodily standards.

Body Image Can Improve as We Age

In a culture like ours, it's difficult to feel comfortable in a female body of any age, much less an aging one. As older women, we not only have to deal with our society's impossible body ideal but also have to contend with all the significant physical losses of the aging process itself. It's hard sometimes not to view our aging bodies with disappointment, fear, or sadness.

The surprising news emerging from large studies of body image across the life span is that our body dissatisfaction does *not* increase with age but tends to stay the same,[15] or even decline a bit.[16] What's more, appearance is considered less important by older women than younger.

The most exciting and unexpected finding, from eminent body image researcher Marika Tiggemann, is that older women actually have higher levels of what's called "body appreciation" than their younger counterparts.[17] Unlike "body dissatisfaction," which assesses negative thoughts and feelings about one's body, "body appreciation" taps the positive dimensions of body image. Body appreciation is defined as accepting, respecting, and having a favorable opinion of one's body, including rejecting unrealistic body ideals portrayed by the media. *More than any other measure of body image, body appreciation is correlated with feelings of well-being.*[18] What is also striking is that you can have elevated scores on both "body appreciation" and "body dissatisfaction." In other words, you can wish your tummy and thighs were smaller at the same time that you maintain an accepting and even favorable sense of your body. In part, this is because we gain more appreciation of our bodies' *abilities* as we get older—for example, our body's ability to stay strong and healthy. In short, even though our bodies diverge further and further from the highly desirable media ideal, we do *not* get more dissatisfied with our bodies as we age. In fact, we appreciate them more. Scientists are beginning to recognize, says Tiggemann, that positive body image gets more complex in older age and that it involves more than the mere absence of body dissatisfaction.

How Body Image Develops

Body image first appears between twenty-five months and thirty-six months of age, when we first recognize our image in the mirror. Most of us then start developing strong beliefs about our bodies in early adolescence, and by the end of the teenage years, these beliefs have solidified into a coherent body image, along with our stereotypes, prejudices, and political attitudes.

When the two-year-old first recognizes herself in the mirror and in the eyes of others, this heralds the beginning of another incredibly important psychological ability, called "self-reflexive" functioning by psychoanalyst Lewis Aron.[19] He defines it as the mental capacity to move back and forth between the view of yourself as a subject ("I") and the view of yourself as an object ("me") seen by others. Your body, particularly your skin surface, plays a huge role in creating this ability to oscillate between subject and object, because your skin is the boundary between me and not-me, inside and outside. People with body image problems, like those with anorexia, have an overdeveloped sense of themselves as "objects" seen by others and have trouble experiencing themselves from the inside, as "I."

According to Self-Objectification Theory,[20] the female body is socially constructed as an object to be looked at and evaluated in our culture. Because women are so often regarded as sexual objects, we learn to look at ourselves from the outside, as critical observers of our own physical appearance. We internalize the "observer" perspective. Then we experience the wish for a more perfect body as our *own* desire, rather than one that has been blasted into us via hundreds of doctored media images a day. We think the problem is in us, in our bodies, not in the fake Photoshopped images offered up to us. (I must add that the male body is also being increasingly objectified, so men are also having more body image problems, though much less so than women.) This kind of heightened self-objectification, studies show, is correlated with body shame, belief in cosmetic surgery, depression, sexual dysfunction, and various forms of disordered eating.

Of course, we all know from personal experience that our body image can shift somewhat from day to day, depending on which pair of jeans we're wearing, what mirror we look in, or what kind of mood we're in. But if we have more significant body image problems, we find ourselves more easily triggered into self-consciousness and negative bodily and mental states. Because we lack an accurate and stable internal image of our body, we must rely on external feedback to help us reconstitute ourselves. When that feedback is negative or critical or overstimulating—"You look different"—our body image can fall apart.

And our body image, because it coalesces so early, remains surprisingly resistant to modification. Sarah Miller, writing in the *New York Times*, gives a heartbreaking account of how persistent body hatred can be, describing herself as "someone whose weight had probably occupied 50 percent of my thinking for my entire life." Most striking is what happened when, as an adolescent, Sarah dieted and lost weight: "People went crazy about my transformation. . . . Every person I talked to now was two people, the one who was nice to me because I was thin, and the person who had been mean to me when I was fat." To this day, she says, "I'm sorry to report that I only like myself thin. . . . At any rate, I'm 50 and I am way too scared of the world to stop dieting. . . . Or at least it is too late for me, and it's too late for pretty much everyone my age. We are so brainwashed. And as imperfect as the body positivity movement may be, just remember: We didn't even have one."[21]

Many people, like my sixteen-year-old patient Chelsea, rely on external images of very thin women to give her "inspiration" to lose weight. She showed me her "very, very favorite image," which she had on her phone and "loved" to look at multiple times a day. It was an image of a young Broadway singer with an impossibly thin waist—so abnormally thin that it was obviously the work of Photoshop surgery. Chelsea believed that this image was a source of motivation to eat less, when actually the photo was eating away at her self-esteem and feeding her eating disorder. Like so many people, she assumed she needed to feel shame about her body in order to "make" her take care of it. In fact, this perspective is out of line with scientific findings, which show that people who appreciate and feel gratitude toward their bodies are *more* likely to take good care of them. Women with a positive body image are more likely to practice intuitive eating, use sun protection, conduct regular breast self-exams, and engage in vigorous exercise—no matter what size their body is.[22]

Having a generally positive body image does not, of course, mean that you love everything about your appearance. No, it suggests that you're not overly concerned with how your body looks. You think of your body more broadly—how it functions, how it allows you to feel pleasure, strength, and vigor and to connect emotionally with people and the world around you. And when you do have negative feelings about your body, you try to give yourself compassion and understanding. If you have a generally positive body image, it fits seamlessly into your imagined view of your external appearance, like a comfortable suit. It is this *broader* sense of body image, with its foundation in strong body awareness, that I am exploring in this book.

Why Women?

Why are we women nine times more likely than men to develop eating disorders, leading some to call them "gendered disorders"? In trying to explain this gender bias, most analyses have focused on our media-saturated culture, with its focus on the "thin ideal." But what happens if we look deeper and earlier into female development?

Since I began treating women with eating disorders over thirty-five years ago, I've been trying to understand more about the particular challenges that women and girls face in our society.[23] While opportunities for females have certainly expanded in the past several decades—girls and women are now allowed to excel in sports, academics, and careers—female bodies are still responded to very differently than male bodies.

Distorted Mirroring

Starting at a very young age, girls' bodies are mirrored by our society in a more distorting and overstimulating manner than boys' are. The girl is encouraged to show off her body, her clothes, her hair, her "smile"—to offer her body for admiration by others. Girls are dressed in little short dresses and tights, always in bright colors and often with sequins, and they do look absolutely darling, and people "ooh" and "ah." The girl often responds by preening and posing and acting coy. The problem is that this kind of intense and often sexualized attention can be "overstimulating" for her. While she may certainly be flattered and pleased, she can also feel *too* "inflated" and too revved up. She may just as easily come crashing down in shame when her displays aren't responded to with delight but, instead, with disregard or criticism. I think of this as the *overstimulation/ shame roller coaster.*

The hormonal and social vicissitudes of adolescence bring further insults to the girl's sense of her bodily self. Girls at this age suddenly learn that from now on they will be expected to behave according to new rules—rules that may seem foreign and incomprehensible. Even if they have nontraditional mothers, girls feel compelled by the sexist media (and its conduit, the "popular" girl) to develop new ways of talking and moving their bodies, their hands, their eyes, and their mouths in order to make themselves "sexy." They are asked to take on a new way of being for which they may feel woefully unequipped. And because girls in today's culture also feel required to show so much skin (even in cold weather!), too many end up feeling overexposed, as they ride the overstimulation/ shame roller coaster.

All of us have a deep and valid human need to be seen and to shine. Women and girls have learned to meet this need through bodily display, because this has been one of the few avenues reliably open to us throughout history. Even as adult women, we are not only allowed but expected to exhibit ourselves. We still attempt to "shine" via our appearance by creating our own eye-catching, creative, flattering, and/ or provocative clothing, makeup, and hairstyles. It can all be quite enjoyable, of course, but my point is that this particular arena of appearance and sexual attractiveness can become *overloaded* for women and girls—not only with expectation and desire, but also with anxiety, conflict, and shame. The girl or woman in our society is left with a confused body—constantly remodeled and decorated to receive admiration, yet always judged and compared and found wanting. It is precisely because females of all ages and time periods have learned to seek recognition and admiration through bodily appearance that we also, I believe, express our distress through *bodily* symptoms and body disorders.

Enter eating disorders, which usually begin around puberty. Body dissatisfaction is invariably present before the onset of an eating disorder. Thus, an eating disorder, despite its name, is, fundamentally a disordered relationship with the *body*, a frantic attempt to manage a sense of bodily vulnerability and the emotional dysregulation that comes with it. As mentioned, women who develop eating disorders tend to have unstable body images and tend to observe themselves more from the outside, rather than experience themselves from the inside.

Mirroring problems also show up in the microcosm of the family. In the early family environment of people with eating disorders, there tends to be an unusual preoccupation with bodily appearance. Mothers of children with eating disorders, studies show, are often preoccupied with their daughters' weight and are more likely to have eating disorders themselves.[24] Unfortunately, these problems tend to get passed down through the female generations. If the mother's body image is unstable, the girl's identification with her mother can result in her having a troubled body image of her own. When she approaches puberty, she can unconsciously experience her maturing body as if her mother's body were being forcibly imposed on her and can attempt to prevent her body from becoming like her mother's by dropping a lot of weight.

Family members often focus on *specific* body parts—for example, the mother of a patient I'll talk about shortly commented on her daughter's "hippo hips." Even when people put too much attention on positive attributes like her "nice long legs," a girl can feel like a collage of isolated body parts. Over time, her body can feel more fragmented and unreal, and she may begin to wall off her body from her total sense of self. This is one reason why people with body image disorders often experience their bodies as alien, separate, out-of-control, hated, "my enemy," and "too much."

I must emphasize at this point that the preoccupation with appearance in society and in the family of origin are not enough to create a body image disorder like an eating disorder. These disorders are *multi*-determined. Sex, age, and social class clearly play a role, as does innate temperament—there is a tendency from the beginning to be more insecure, driven, and perfectionistic. For anorexia to be triggered in the first place, you must experience a significant drop in weight, which might be the result of, say, a sudden "growth spurt," an illness, or the competitive pressures of a team sport. And there are many other important reasons why women can feel alienated from their bodies, which I mentioned in chapter 3, including extreme dysmenorrhea, shame about breasts being "too big" or "too small," and physical or sexual abuse.

Competing Female Role Demands

Many studies show that women with body image problems tend to overidentify with the female role, including the need to be caretaking, perfect, and slim.[25] Our amazing Olympic women's soccer team notwithstanding, girls and women can still feel reticent about behaving assertively or aggressively in the classroom or boardroom or at a dinner party, at the same time that they are expected to be successful at work, then confidently take on the "second shift" at home as supermom. Girls and women are still expected to moderate their own feelings of expansiveness and assertiveness if they are perceived to be in conflict with the needs of others, and it may be that becoming thinner is a way of making oneself "smaller" in every way except caregiving. Taking care of others is still the overarching role assigned to women, and, in this arena (as with appearance), women are allowed, even encouraged, to shine or excel.

At the same time, we of the Boomer generation and those following have been offered more and more opportunities to take on traditionally male roles of breadwinner, professional, artist, expert, or leader. It is probably not a coincidence that women started trying harder to get thinner in the 1970s at the same time that the birth control pill allowed us to delay marriage and childrearing and enter the labor force in greater numbers and in higher-paying jobs.[26] It can be argued that as women got more successful outside the home, they felt the need to become more androgynous—becoming thinner and less curvy and, in the late 1980s, even adding huge shoulder pads to "power up" and take more of the weight of the world on our shoulders. We Boomers, and to some degree members of the next cohort, Generation X, grew up "betwixt and between" the old order and the new, so that, if we were at home raising kids, we could feel ambivalent about being in the traditional female role, or, if we were in the outside workforce, we could feel ambivalent about our nontraditional roles. We have always found ourselves juggling competing and often conflicting role aspirations and demands—and, I would argue, our body images have had trouble keeping up.

Gina

I would now like to tell you more about my forty-nine-year-old patient Gina, whom I introduced at the top of this chapter. Gina, who had always struggled with her weight and her body image, came from an outwardly stable, "normal," middle-class home. Her mother, however, was obsessed by Gina's weight, particularly what she called Gina's "hippo hips," and put Gina on her first Metrical diet when she was ten. Gina's mother also picked out Gina's clothes for her until she was twenty-seven years old, and they were always dark-colored, slimming, and "sensible." A striking example of her mother's confusion of her own needs with her daughter's was when she told Gina, "For my birthday, all I want is for *you* to lose weight." Gina's attempts to "shine" in other ways were also discounted; for example, her parents never attended her school performances.

Gina came into treatment at the urgent recommendation of her physician, because she had lost over thirty-five pounds in less than five months and was descending into dangerously low-weight territory. Gina, however, was loving it. She thought she looked great, especially the way she looked in clothes. Losing the weight had remobilized her thwarted childhood need to be seen and delighted in, and she had begun buying clothes compulsively and exhibiting herself proudly to all those around her, including me. When she walked into my office, she would check out my outfit and then adjust her own posture as if expecting me to be checking her out as well.

Shopping became the main focus of Gina's life. She would shop at consignment and retail stores three times a week, saying she was afraid of "missing something." She described in great detail the incredible "high" of trying on clothes in her favorite store and getting "oohs and ahs" from the clerks. Before long, there were dozens of bags of clothes in her closet, some unopened. The shopping had become an addiction.

Each morning, Gina would deliberate for an hour or more about what outfit to wear, sometimes making herself late to work. Her indecision about what to wear paralleled her struggle with her body image. What image did she want to project? What clothes made her feel better? What did she want to express about herself that day? Who would be seeing her that day? One respected male and one respected female coworker loomed particularly large in her fantasies of being admired.

On the positive side, her experimentation with clothing was allowing her to play with her body image in new and creative ways. For the first time in her life, she felt attractive. Creating a sense of a proud and beautiful self through clothing was a way to differentiate herself from her mother's critical view of her body. I could well understand how wonderful it felt to *finally* be getting some admiring responses from those around her, and my own interest in and quiet delight in her new clothing pizzazz provided some of the early mirroring of her body self that she had so sorely missed. Of course, *my* body was also a part of the treatment; in her imagination, I could enjoy looking good as well as enjoy food and sex. I also tried to keep an unswerving focus on the health of her body, including her eating, and over time, her weight stabilized at a not super-thin but normal level.

Because she had finally gotten some of the affirmation that she had sorely needed as a child to build her body self, Gina found herself with a sense of having a more "real" body—specifically, a real female body—which was feeling more like an integral part of herself. Gina started talking with me about her lifelong relationship with her body: "This body has never been okay. I always felt trapped in this body. I hated this body. When my body wanted things, I always told it, 'No, you're just a body!'" She hadn't accepted that her "wanting" body was a part of "her," because her parents couldn't meet her wants and she knew it. Rather than try to get what she needed and fail, she took a safer route and walled off her body, making it "this body," not "my body."

As time went on, I talked with her more about how she didn't seem to be aware of her *inner* body, her body's sensations and desires. I noted that she was much more conscious of the body that other people *see* than the body she herself *feels*. We talked in much more detail about her very poor and sporadic eating and about how she would walk around in horribly uncomfortable shoes all day long that left her feet blistered and bruised. I encouraged her to be kind to her body, her poor body, which had been so neglected, criticized, and controlled when she was growing up. I encouraged her to tune into her "inside body." One day she told me rather shyly that she'd discovered that she felt happier and less anxious when she was being "nice" to her body and when she wasn't only thinking about how she looked. Gina was beginning to move inward, into experiencing her body from the inside and outside at the same time. Her body was beginning to feel more like her own.

Interoceptive Awareness as an Ageism Disruptor

I've been focusing in this chapter mainly on body image, but our experience of our body has two fundamental components: *body image* and *interoception*. Body image relates to our internal *picture* of our body, while interoception refers to our internal *feeling* of our body. Together, they provide the foundation of our sense of personal identity and overall well-being.

And it turns out that body image and interoception are powerfully interrelated. Interoception, as you've learned, is the ongoing processing and mapping of your internal somatic sensations, which is responsible for maintaining your homeostasis, the physiological condition of your body. And you know that a wide range of body experiences—your self-awareness, your emotional life, your sense of body ownership, your sense of agency—are also shaped by the interoceptive process. But only recently are major neuroscientists like Manos Tsakiris and Olga Pollatos looking at how *interoception influences body image*, and the results are exciting. Evidence from both neuroimaging and questionnaire research is revealing that people with higher interoceptive awareness—a greater ability to sense internal body signals—have a more accurate and stable body image and greater bodily satisfaction.[27] In fact, having good interoceptive awareness appears to be a necessary condition for a strong body image. Without a well-developed *sense* of your body, your body image will not feel real and will be more of an abstract, often inaccurate, idea of who you are.

The brain circuits that make up your body image are spread widely throughout your brain, wherever beliefs are stored. Like all beliefs, beliefs about your body arise in response to your brain's ongoing predictions about how the world operates. This helps explain why, for example, after you lose twenty-five pounds, you still feel overweight: the expectation of being fat that is lodged in your brain is still traveling back down the cortical hierarchy and into the body, making your body still feel fat! This is true of all kinds of body transformations, as, for example, when you become more muscular or more limber through yoga. When such change occurs, your body image must slowly adjust to conform to your actual physical body. Intentionally developing your body awareness can help you keep mind and body better aligned.

A distorted and unstable body image, like Gina's, is a core feature of eating disorders, particularly anorexia. Anorexic individuals view their severely underweight bodies as normal or even large and are constantly driven to lose weight. This is because people with anorexia are less able to register interoceptive sensations related to hunger and fullness.[28] Brain imaging studies show reduced activity in the insula, which suggests lower self-awareness in general, including a diminished ability to "follow your gut" or your heart.[29] It follows, therefore, that women with reduced levels of interoceptive awareness are more likely to treat themselves as objects, to look at themselves from the outside rather than the inside—as described in Self-Objectification Theory. Lowered interoceptive awareness, as I've mentioned, is also found in other disorders involving disturbed body image, like self-harm disorders, depression, obesity, and schizophrenia.

The findings on "body ownership" add another important piece to our understanding of interoception and body image. You will recall that "body ownership" is the sense that your body sensations, movements, and body parts are uniquely your own and will not be confused with anyone else's. Neuroscientists studying body ownership use various clever means to trick a subject into thinking that her hand is not really her hand or her face not her face—like the Rubber Hand Illusion I described earlier. In the "enfacement illusion," a participant is synchronously touched on the same part of the face as another person standing in front of her; she has the illusion of looking at her *own* face in a mirror when, in fact, she is looking at the other person's face. Individuals with lower interoceptive awareness, studies show, are more vulnerable to losing their sense of body ownership in response to certain external stimuli.[30]

In other words, the less aware you are of your internal sensations, the more influenced you will be by external stimuli, which deepens our understanding of why some women are more prone than others to overidentify with media images of young, slim, perfected female bodies. This research makes it clear how deepening our body awareness can help us resist the insidious visual brainwashing of our ageist society.

Moving from Outside to Inside

So, we've all grown up under the "male gaze" in our ageist, image-saturated culture. Our bodies have been mirrored back to us in distorted, confusing, and overstimulating ways, and we've taken on challenging new roles with competing role demands. We have also learned to dismiss or hate or feel ashamed of our bodies for many other reasons, related to family and subcultural norms and prejudices, or physical or emotional inheritance, or traumatic experiences.

But we cannot ignore that other crucial reason for our widespread body insecurity, which is still largely unrecognized and is the focus of this book: we have never really gotten to know our bodies, to sense and feel our bodies from the inside out. "Growing up" in our culture meant giving up that in-the-moment somatic awareness we had as babies in favor of cognitive adroitness. We never really learned to read and interpret sensations arising from within our bodies and to use this information to make decisions about what we need and want. The result, as I've suggested, is a mind-body disconnect that keeps us from knowing ourselves deeply. This is particularly dangerous for us as we age, when we become more physically vulnerable and need to take even better care of our precious bodies.

So how do we begin to rewrite these body-hating, body-dismissing narratives and instead make friends with our aging bodies? How can we resist and counter our society's obsession with appearance and youth? How can we push back against our culture's preoccupation with being youthfully smart, "quick," "on"? My suggestion (of course!) is to *focus inward*: focus on how your body feels from the inside, rather than how it looks from the outside. Focus on the sensation of your body as a whole. Like Gina, we feel so much happier and more relaxed when we stop envisioning the body that others see—the one we think is too fat, too wrinkled, or too saggy—and allow ourselves to enjoy the body we sense and feel and that keeps us alive and kicking. We feel so much stronger when we pay more attention to the "inside body."

Our interoceptive pathways, as you now know, are constantly picking up information from inside and outside our bodies and making emotional predictions, through complex computations, to figure out what we need to do *right now* to maintain our physical and emotional equilibrium. If we also consciously listen to our bodies, we can better use this emotional information to take good care of ourselves. Only by being fully aware of our "inside bodies" in the present moment can we *fix* things that may be going awry—like stretching out that tight neck that's making us feel so tense. It's never too late to start. It's certainly not a question of either/or—we want to enjoy our bodies *both* inside and out. We can enjoy looking good and being fit while remaining aware of our whole-body sensations and feelings.

Checking in with Your Body

I had a revelation around age sixty-five that I could best negotiate many challenges of aging by *starting with my body*. I was finding that so many everyday issues—like low energy, anxiety, stiffness, fatigue, weakness, uncertainty, feeling "old," as well as injury—could be diminished by very simply relaxing or energizing my body through breathing, stretching, or strengthening my muscles. But there is a crucial first step, and this is to *check in with your body*. How else can you know what you need?

As you get up in the morning, do you check in with your body? How is your body feeling this morning? Relaxed? Stiff? Lethargic? What does it need? Or do you immediately start making a to-do list for the day or search for things to worry about? As you drink your morning coffee, can you really taste and smell that coffee? Or are you skimming the newspaper with all brain cells firing and letting in no sensory information? Can you, as Zen Buddhism teaches, *just drink* your coffee without needing to do anything else or think about anything else? As you walk to the car, can you *just walk*? How good it feels to just be present in this moment with this body at this time in this place. Older age, with its wider time perspective, offers us an expansive new opportunity to let go of our monkey brains and return to our bodies. There is no better time to slow down and feel.

Do you spend as much time in *nature* as possible, hopefully every day? As you walk through that glade of trees, can you deliberately move your awareness to the sounds entering your ears—the rustling of the aspen, the chirping of the sparrow?—which magically brings you smack into the moment and into incredible pleasure? I think one reason we love watching our dogs romping on the beach or our cats slowly stretching themselves in the sun is because animals *really* know how to enjoy their bodies. They show us an "other" way of being, a path of body delight that we lost when we were children and we've been grieving for and hungering to return to ever since. Spending time in nature also reminds you that you too are part of the natural cycle of life, a crucial realization for aging with equanimity.

And I must clarify that being broadly aware of our body sensations does not mean that we obsess or worry about every tingle or ache in a way that can become hypochondriacal, which does happen with some older people. No, we want to live as comfortably in our bodies as we can, and, as I say throughout the book, staying aware of our bodies is exactly what we need in order to feel *less* worried and more vital, grounded, and in charge of ourselves as we age. As you learned in previous chapters, having higher body awareness means having more emotional control, greater decisiveness, and a stronger sense of self. Developing body awareness is not, therefore, "soft" or "woo-woo." It is literally the foundation of every kind of strength and power—whether that of a mother, artist, grandmother, teacher, entrepreneur, or politician running for president. If you're truly aware of your body, it feels crazy to ignore, "override," or mistreat your body. It's harder to say, "Oh, who cares, it's just my body" when you really grasp that, in fact, your body is *you*.

I passionately believe that we must feel comfortable *in* our aging body before we can feel comfortable *with* our aging body. As you move through the second half or third of your life, you have a golden opportunity to reconnect mind and body—to become embodied. You can learn to sense and feel your body more, including your body as a whole. In this way, you can keep on revising your sense of your body and self until the very end. The burgeoning new body science helps counter our culture's fear of aging, instead transforming our vision of who we can be as we get older. We'll get to that in the chapters to come. In the meantime, try the following practice for greater self-acceptance and appreciation.

Self-Guided Exercise: Study Your Face

The purpose of this exercise is to help you discover and embody your natural, unique, older beauty.

- Seat yourself comfortably, holding a good, clear hand mirror.

- Looking at yourself in the mirror, study your face deeply and carefully for at least two minutes.

- What do you see in your face? What emotions? Life experience? Character traits? What else? (Take notes or record what you see.)

- What do you find particularly appealing or interesting about your face?

- Having looked deeply into your face, what would you now like to say to yourself that communicates understanding, acceptance, and love?

Chapter 6

Building Body Awareness

A few days after arriving in New Delhi in 1975, my husband and I struggled through shouting and shoving crowds to climb aboard a filthy third-class bus, then a train, to travel nonstop, upright, for two days and nights to Manali, a beautiful village in the Kulu Valley, high in the Himalayas. We were there to do a meditation retreat with a Theravadan Buddhist monk named Luong Pi (now Christopher Titmuss, a meditation teacher in England). We moved into an empty house, perched on the edge of a cliff, with twenty-five or so other Westerners—the women sleeping side-by-side on the floor in one room, the men in another. For the next ten days, we would arise at 3:30 a.m., do sun salutations on the deck, then hourlong sitting meditation followed by walking meditation, a breakfast of oatmeal and prunes, then meditation instruction, and more meditation until a one-bowl vegetarian main meal at midday, then more meditation, a short time for chores, and more meditation. There was no supper, only a cup of tea and two biscuits, followed by a dharma talk by Luong Pi, then more meditation, and, finally, sleep at 10 p.m. The kind of meditation we were doing was Vipassana, or "Insight" meditation, and most of it involved focusing on our breath or "sweeping" the body with our attention, noticing any internal and external body sensations like tingling, hunger, tightness, pain, numbness, throbbing, pleasure, itching, or pressure. We were meditating about twelve hours a day—more if we felt like it, which I sometimes did. After that first retreat, we decided to stay for another, then another, finally spending an entire month in almost continuous meditation. I will never forget the day we left the retreat and took a taxi to the bus station. What before had seemed chaotic, cacophonous, and overwhelming now felt like "just the way things are." The pushing and shouting hardly fazed me. My body and mind were clear. Negotiating the station now seemed simple, because I was finally really paying attention. I was suffused with a quiet joy. Something inside me had broken open, and I had moved into a completely different state of being. I had achieved (for a little while) what Buddhists called "equanimity."

Meditating twelve hours a day for a month in ascetic conditions is not, of course, for everyone—and wouldn't be for me now. It was a particular moment in history, when the "counterculture" arose out of a protest movement and spawned the Woodstock generation, and when tens of thousands of young people flocked to India to study with meditation masters, following in the footsteps of Harvard professors turned gurus . . . and the Beatles! Even before going to India, when I was working as a journalist and then a doctoral student in psychology, I had been attending various meditation talks and groups and keeping a little meditation practice going.

But none of that had prepared me for the experience I had on the mountaintop in India, which was the result of sustained, lengthy daily practice. This is validated by the explosion of research on meditation over the past two decades, which I will summarize shortly. Studies show that you gain significant benefit from even small amounts of meditation practice, especially in the realm of emotional regulation and stress relief, and that the benefits just keep building as your meditative practice gets more stable, regular, and sustained. If you happen to be in that small slice of the populace that gravitates toward more intense meditation training—five-day, ten-day, three-month retreats—you may have a transformative experience. Indeed, scientists are now studying people at the extreme end of meditative practice, described by leading neuroscientific researcher Richard Davidson in his terrific book *Altered Traits*, written with Daniel Goleman.[1] At his lab at the University of Wisconsin, Davidson studies "Olympic-level" Tibetan yogis who have permanently transformed their minds—their neural circuitry, their brain waves—through meditation, as I'll describe later.

I am so grateful that the stars somehow aligned and I got to that mountaintop in India, because I learned at a young age the power of being in my body. My knowledge of that profoundly embodied state never really left me, even during the intervening decades, as I was knocked around by our speedy, conceptual society while building my career, raising a child, and caring for my declining mother. I lived for too many years with too much anxiety and too many hands-like-hooks pulling me in too many directions. Yet I never completely forgot what I learned in Manali. When I did manage to sit on the cushion or lie on the mat or make it to a meditation retreat, I could often still get back to that spacious room inside me.

After menopause, free from all those hormones and responsibilities, I found my body quieter inside, and I finally started slowing down. When I turned sixty, it really hit me that I was in the last third of my life—that there was a lot less time ahead and much more behind.[2] I found myself naturally feeling more protective of my body and mind, which I knew would be getting less robust and would need more attention and care. It felt crazy not to do everything I could to take good care of myself as I grew older. I wanted to slide into older age in the best health possible. That's when I began to delve into the science and practice of body awareness.

The practices for building internal body awareness have different names—like meditation, yoga, tai chi, breath work—but I don't really consider them separate entities, because, as scholars are continuing to discover, they are all forms of meditation that work in large part by promoting interoceptive awareness.

Contemplative Practices and Interoception

Hundreds of scientists around the world are currently studying ancient, mainly Buddhist "contemplative practices." The Dalai Lama lit this flame in 2001 when he invited leading scientists from several Western countries to his palace in Dharamsala, India, to discuss "destructive emotions." At the end of the meetings, this revered Buddhist leader asked Davidson, who was one of the scientists, "Why can't you use the same tools from modern neuroscience to study kindness and compassion that you use for studying anxiety and fear and depression and stress?" That question became the guiding inspiration for Davidson and many other scientists to turn toward the investigation of positive emotions and how best to cultivate them.

Twenty years later, in May 2021, this original meeting was reprised in the online Science and Wisdom of Emotions Summit,[3] which brought together the Dalai Lama and other Buddhist masters with leading Western scientists to discuss best practices for training emotional well-being, emotional intelligence, and compassion. The online audience totaled 190,000 people! The idea of global compassion—the ability to have compassion for all beings on the planet, not just for loved ones or oneself—emerged as the summit's shining aspiration. Earlier, in 2015, a different group of researchers from around the world had come together at the University of California Medical Center in San Francisco to share and integrate *interoceptive* research findings and wisdom from both Eastern and Western traditions.

What the Eastern contemplative and Western scientific approaches have in common is the conviction that awareness of *embodied experience* is crucial for well-being and, further, that the ability to have such awareness can be trained. All agree that an overdependence on conceptual awareness, in contrast to sensory awareness, significantly limits a human being's potential for relating meaningfully to self, others, and the world. It's also now clear that embodied awareness must be actively maintained, cultivated, and renewed to sustain our sense of well-being.

Western researchers, like Norman Farb at the University of California, San Francisco (UCSF), are finding concepts in the contemplative traditions that are remarkably similar to those arising out of the Western science of interoception—for example, the concept of the "subtle body," with its "subtle energies" (*chi* in Mandarin, *prana* in Sanskrit, and *lung* in Tibetan) flowing through "channels," "meridians," and "chakras."[4] These "energy flows" have been an important focus of Chinese, Indian, and Tibetan medicine for millennia, and it is not yet clear how they map onto the Western science of interoception and its applications. I must also note that modern practices of mindfulness are not equivalent to traditional practices. Popular modern practices, like Jon Kabat-Zinn's Mindfulness-Based Stress Reduction (MBSR), aim to reduce emotional distress, while classical traditions seek nothing less than insight into the fundamental nature of reality and the liberation of the human mind from its conditioning. I hope to show you how many meditative practices, ancient and modern, not only can relieve emotional distress but also can help liberate us from our conditioning, including conditioning that rules how we live in our aging bodies.

A Prediction Machine

Basically, your brain is a prediction machine, constantly appraising your body sensations, then creating simulations to predict what will happen next. These simulations, or neural maps of your body at higher and higher levels of your brain, are a best approximation of your body's current state, as predicted by prior states, from which you can interpret your experience and coordinate your actions.

Your brain is constantly comparing your *sensed* bodily state to your body as you *expect* it to be, based on your prior experiences.[5] You are constantly trying to resolve the tension created by the discrepancy between your "sensed" versus "expected" bodily state. If there is a mismatch between your current sensed and expected states, you can do either of two things: (1) you can try to change your current sensation to meet your expected state ("active inference"), or (2) you can adjust your expected state to match your current sensation ("perceptual inference"). Here's an example: let's say you go outside and find it uncomfortably hot; you could drink an ice-cold glass of water to change your body temperature, or, alternatively, you could decide to welcome the hot weather and relax and enjoy it.

Of course, your ongoing attitude toward your internal sensations, which you have been developing all your life, may powerfully affect which of these two approaches you will prefer. For example, when you feel too hot, is that feeling associated in your mind with how miserable and short-tempered your dad would get when *he* was too hot when you were a child? If that's the case, you'll probably try to get away from that "hot" sensation as quickly as you can.

Top-Down Versus Bottom-Up

These two strategies for dealing with body states can be boiled down into a "doing versus being" approach to life's challenges, which can also translate into "Western versus Eastern" or "top-down versus bottom-up." In top-down regulation, we use our "higher" thinking brain to control our "lower" bodily states; in bottom-up regulation, we pay attention to and accept what is actually happening in our body.

Some Western psychological therapies, like Cognitive Behavioral Therapy, emphasize changing negative thoughts, an example of "top-down" regulation in which we use our "higher" brain to regulate our "lower" body states. Contemplative traditions, like meditation or yoga, promote "bottom-up" strategies, like acceptance or noninterfering observation of our bodily experience (as do some contemporary Western psychological therapies, like Dialectical Behavior Therapy and Acceptance and Commitment Therapy). In fact, contemplative teachers often argue that attempting to control or regulate emotional/bodily experience is itself the problem. In eating disorders, for example, people often turn to food to solve every kind of problem, whether it be stress, anger, or loneliness, a kind of active or top-down strategy that works only temporarily. In modern Western culture in general, the balance has shifted into the "doing" mode. We go for quick fixes for anything that ails us, like having a drink or looking at funny animal videos on Facebook. Bottom-up approaches tend to be less intuitive for us, unless we are specifically taught to cultivate certain attentional abilities, intentions, and attitudes.[6]

The aim of mindfulness practices and mindfulness-based therapies is to encourage a transition from "doing" to "being"—to increase "bottom-up" attention to what is actually happening in the body rather than attempting to alter body sensations to fit "top-down" expectations of what *should* happen in the body. Only then can we harness the excellent and necessary information residing in our body sensations, information that lets us know more deeply how we *are* and what we *need*. Focusing attention on our actual bodily sensations rather than on mental appraisals of them also allows us to stop and observe before acting—so we don't, for example, automatically respond to unpleasant things with avoidance or to pleasure with approach. Becoming more aware of our body states also helps us move away from the unhealthy process of rumination, in which we obsessively, repetitively "chew on" negative concerns.

Presence and Agency

As we become more embodied, two incredibly important abilities arise: (1) *presence*, your connection to the present moment, and (2) *agency*, your ability to bring about change.[7] Both are foundations of your sense of well-being. Presence is a feeling of engagement with your body and your environment, the direct and intense experience of the here and now. Agency is a feeling of control over your actions in the world, a sense that you can be effective, influence your life, and assume responsibility for your behavior. (Your sense of agency, however, should not be confused with "top-down" regulation, because with agency you remain grounded in your actual body sensations, rather than trying to revise them.) Both agency and presence are vital for self-regulation; in fact, agency makes you *responsible* for self-regulation, giving you the impetus, for example, to monitor your breath when anxious or to quit a stressful job. It gives you the confidence to remain grounded, yet flexible and resilient, in the face of conflict or change. You can see that presence and agency tend to co-occur. You must be *present* and connected to your body and environment in order to determine the best action to take.

I must point out that feeling one's visceral sensations may sometimes be distressing, even harmful, for people prone to panic, PTSD, or other anxiety disorders. They may "catastrophize" interoceptive signals—thinking, for example, "my heart is beating wildly, I must be having a heart attack." With the right meditative instruction, however, such people can learn to revise their interpretations of their internal signals. Women with a history of interpersonal sexual violence, research shows, can learn to register when sensory cues to dissociate ("space out") get triggered, which allows them to maintain awareness of their bodies instead of moving into their habitual, fearful "top-down" regulatory responses. Over time, these women discover that their body can be an informative resource rather than a source of threat, so they can feel safer in the world, more able to engage in intimate interactions with their spouse/partner, and more grounded, agentic, and empowered.[8] If you find yourself blocking your body sensations for fear of triggering frightening emotions, seek out an excellent trauma-trained psychotherapist who can, ideally, collaborate in your treatment with an excellent trauma-trained body worker.

Practices for Strengthening Embodiment

Let's now look more closely at different body practices—meditation, breathing, yoga, tai chi/qigong, chanting, and others. We will consider the "how to," science, and benefits of each, and how they can help us as we age. All include the same basic ingredients—breathing, meditation, and movement/nonmovement. I start with mindfulness meditation only because it is far and away the most studied practice.

Mindfulness Meditation

Mindfulness is the practice of returning, again and again, to the present moment. This is true when practicing mindfulness meditation or when practicing mindfulness while doing the dishes. I will mainly present the Vipassana style of Buddhist meditation, which began in southeast Asia, since it is the focus of most of the research and what I am most familiar with.

In the beginning form of Vipassana mindfulness meditation, often called *focused attention,* you focus on the in-and-out-breath as an anchor to the present moment. As your mind wanders—which is what minds do—you have to bring your awareness back to your breath again and again. Using brain scans, neuroscientists are able to observe when the meditator becomes *distracted* (in the "default-mode network," which is particularly active when the brain is in a state of wakeful rest), when the meditator becomes *aware* of the distraction (in the brain's "salience network," which selects which stimuli deserve our attention), and when the focus on the breath is *restored* (in the dorsolateral prefrontal cortex).[9]

If you don't already have your own basic meditation practice, try this:

Set aside some time and space—ten minutes is enough to begin with.

Sit comfortably. If on a cushion, cross your legs comfortably in front of you. If on a chair, rest the bottoms of your feet on the floor or on a cushion so that your legs are not dangling.

Straighten your upper body, but don't stiffen. Let your posture be relaxed.

Rest the palms of your hands on your legs wherever they feel comfortable.

Soften your gaze. Drop your chin a little and let your gaze fall gently downward. Let whatever appears before your eyes be there without focusing on it.

Bring your attention to the physical sensation of breathing. Gently focus on the air moving through your nose or mouth, or the rising and falling of your belly or your chest.

Observe the present moment as it is. Simply pay attention to the present moment, without judgment.

When you notice your mind wandering, gently return your attention to your breath.

Be kind to yourself if you find your mind wandering constantly. This is normal. Come back to your breath over and over again, without judgment or expectation.

When you're ready to end, gently lift your gaze. Take a moment to notice any sounds, and slowly move your body back and forth to help you come back to your surroundings. Notice how your body feels now.

With more experience, you can progress to what is called "open-monitoring" mindfulness, which involves simply noticing sights, sounds, thoughts, and sensations, including internal bodily sensations, without a particular attentional focus on your breath.

Other Forms of Meditation

In addition to basic mindfulness, you can try other forms of meditation to vary your routine. All are extremely useful. While they all incorporate aspects of mindfulness, they also offer alternative foci of attention.

Loving Kindness (Metta in Sanskrit)

The aim of this form of meditation, which was made popular by Vipassana teacher Sharon Salzberg,[10] is to feel compassion for yourself and others.

> Focus on yourself and, for ten minutes or so, send positive thoughts to yourself, saying slowly over and over, "May you be happy. May you be healthy. May you be safe. May you live with ease."
>
> Think of someone you love or who is special in your life and send these wishes to her or him.
>
> Think of someone who is "difficult" or "aversive" for you and send these wishes to her or him.

You can also send loving kindness to strangers, to "benefactors," or to animals. The possibilities are endless. Different teachers suggest different wordings for this practice, and sometimes you are encouraged to come up with your own phrases, which convey the same sorts of kind and loving wishes. Here is a special version of metta for aging comfortably[11]:

> As I grow older, may I be kind to myself.
>
> As I grow older, may I accept joy and sorrow.
>
> As I grow older, may I be happy and at peace.

When I was first introduced to loving kindness meditation, I, like many people, found it kind of hokey and not as "pure" as silent meditation. But what I have since learned from the research is that it is one of the most powerful forms of meditation there is. Studies show that metta meditation dramatically builds empathy and compassion, helps improve self-esteem, and even helps resolve conflicts with others. It is particularly effective in treating post-traumatic stress disorder. Not surprisingly, the brain regions involved in empathy that I described earlier—like the insula and the anterior cingulate cortex, as well as the temporoparietal junction—light up during loving kindness meditation.[12]

Walking Meditation

During walking meditation, you focus on each step as you very slowly and mindfully lift and place each foot on the ground. When your mind wanders off into thought, you simply return it to the sensation of your feet on the ground. You can walk anywhere—a hallway indoors, a sidewalk in the city, a path in a park. On meditation retreats, walking meditation is often alternated with sitting meditation to relieve, strengthen, and stretch out the body. It offers the same advantages as sitting meditation.

Body Scan

In this popular form of meditation, you focus on all your bodily sensations, not just your breath. Popularized by MBSR founder Kabat-Zinn[13] and included in many forms of yoga, it is particularly effective when led by a teacher.

> Lying on your back on the floor, very slowly scan your whole body, noticing any sensations—tightness, prickles, tickles, numbness, pain, and so on. Starting with your toes, slowly move your attention up through your legs and on to your pelvis, buttocks, abdomen, chest, shoulders, arms, neck, head, ears, parts of your face, and top of your head. Areas like your abdomen, shoulders, jaws, and eyes, which hold a lot of tension, may need particular attention.

Body scan meditation is particularly good at reducing anxiety or stress and managing chronic pain and for building interoceptive awareness. You can find Kabat-Zinn leading body-scan meditation on YouTube.

If you haven't done meditation before, it's important to start slowly. Ten minutes a day is fine; then, if you feel like it, ten minutes twice a day, or twenty minutes once a day. Some people immediately take to it and want to do more—that's fine too. Don't be discouraged if meditation feels somewhat uncomfortable, or boring, or strange at first. There's no "right" way to feel. You don't have to stop thinking to meditate. Just notice whatever thoughts and feelings come up.

The Benefits of Meditation

The booming meditation field is filled with enough exaggerated claims to make anyone skeptical, so I will briefly highlight only major findings that have been confirmed by neuroimaging and/or replicated in many studies.

- **Increased interoceptive awareness:** Meditation helps anchor your attention to your breath and other internal body sensations. People report feeling more aware of their bodies on the Multidimensional Assessment of Interoceptive Awareness (MAIA),[14] and brain scans show more activation in major brain regions for interoceptive processing.[15] However, a study by Sahib Khalsa shows conclusively that meditation does not increase interoceptive heartbeat detection, but, interestingly, that meditators do report experiencing heartbeat sensations more widely throughout the body than nonmeditators.[16]

- **Emotion regulation:** The most heralded and sturdy finding across thousands of studies is that meditation, practiced over time periods ranging from days to months, helps you regulate your emotions and react less to stress, both of which boost your sense of well-being.[17]

- **Sharpened attention:** Even short amounts of meditation increase your brain's ability to focus on one thing and ignore distractions[18] as well as enhancing your readiness to respond to new stimuli. Gains from more intensive meditation can even last seven years or more.

- **Compassion:** You can significantly and rather quickly increase your capacity for compassion—that is, the recognition of and concern for the suffering of others—through meditation, particularly "loving kindness" (*metta*) meditation.[19]

- **"Treatment" for depression and anxiety:** Meditation can decrease depression (particularly severe depression), anxiety, and pain about as much as medication but with no side effects and less relapse.[20] Mindfulness meditation combined with cognitive therapy (Mindfulness-Based Cognitive Therapy) is the most empirically proven psychological treatment with a meditation basis. *However, if your doctor or psychiatrist has prescribed medication for you, do not stop taking it on your own and substitute meditation. If you are considering changing or stopping your medication, you must discuss it with your doctor first.*

"Olympic" Meditators

We can sometimes best understand the power of a human activity like meditation by looking at its extremes, because then we can see what's possible. Mingyur Rinpoche, a forty-one-year-old Tibetan meditation master and teacher, had meditated more than sixty-two thousand hours, including ten full years on retreat, when neuroscientist Davidson and his team asked if he would be willing to have his brain studied. In the first session, they hooked Mingyur up to an electroencephalogram (EEG) machine and asked him to practice meditation to specifically generate *compassion* for sixty seconds, rest for thirty seconds, then repeat the cycle three more times. As soon as he started meditating, the research team was stunned by the dramatic surge of electrical signal that appeared on the computer screens. Each time that Mingyur was signaled to meditate, the computers burst with a wild display of "high-amplitude gamma," the most intense form of EEG frequency. In Davidson and Goleman's words, "The lab team knew at that moment they were witnessing something profound, something that had never before been observed in the laboratory. None could predict what this would lead to, but everyone sensed this was a critical inflection point in neuroscience history."[21]

When Mingyur meditated, fMRI images showed that his internal neural circuitry for empathy jumped in activity by 700 to 800 percent. What fascinated Davidson most was that his team had beginning evidence that a heightened state experienced in meditation could become a lasting *trait*, a permanent part of one's being. Since then, they have studied dozens of these "Olympic-level meditators" and found the same distinctive neural pattern when meditating. Gamma, the very fastest brain wave, occurs when differing brain regions fire in harmony. Astonishingly, this sustained gamma pattern goes on even when seasoned meditators are asleep, another proof that the neural transformations arising out of years of meditation are enduring: that they are genuine "altered traits."

Can Meditation Help Us Age?

As we age, our thought processes begin to slow down as our brain volume very gradually decreases about 5 percent per decade from the age of thirty-five through age sixty and then decreases faster after age seventy. Much of this reduction in volume comes from the shrinking of the prefrontal cortex and hippocampus. The prefrontal cortex is what we use to set goals, make plans, exercise impulse control, and decide what to pay attention to, and as it slows, we find it more difficult to keep track of thoughts (*What did I want to get from the kitchen?*) and to prevent stray thoughts from interfering. And the gradual shrinkage of the hippocampus makes storing and retrieving memories more difficult. (*What's the name of that actor in, um, you know, that movie um, by that director, um . . . ?*) A reduction in the electrical connectivity between our brain cells also leads to a general slowing of mental processes, due in part to a thinning of the myelin sheath, which insulates our neurons and makes them fire faster.

You'll remember from chapter 3 that our interoceptive abilities decline with age, but that, with increased experience, we can do more with the internal sensations we have. Well, one thing we can *do* about various aging difficulties is *meditation*. The research on meditation looks promising for us! Following are some of the research findings.

Younger "Biological Age"

Several encouraging studies of older meditators show that their "biological age" is younger than that of nonmeditators. One of the earliest respected studies on Transcendental Meditation in the early 1980s found that people who had been practicing meditation for more than five years had "biomarkers" (like levels of DHEA hormone) twelve years younger than their chronical age.[22]

More recently, University of California, Los Angeles, researcher Eileen Luders and her team looked at age-related gray-matter atrophy using a special algorithm and found that the brains of fifty longtime meditators were "younger" by 7.5 years than the brains of nonmeditators of the same age.[23] And when Sara Lazar, mentioned in chapter 1, analyzed her meditator subjects for age effects, she was surprised to find that fifty-year-old meditators had as much gray matter in their brains as twenty-five-year-olds, suggesting that meditation and yoga may slow down the age-related atrophy of the prefrontal cortex, which controls executive functioning, and the hippocampus, specialized for memory.[24]

Davidson has also found that the brains of those master meditators he is studying are aging more slowly. He has scanned Mingyur Rinpoche's brain periodically for two decades, comparing his brain to norms for his age, and finds him in the ninety-ninth percentile—the youngest in a group of 100 matched peers. At the age of forty-one, Mingyur had the brain of someone more like thirty-three.[25] Davidson's lab has repeated these findings with a larger group of super-meditators. While you or I are not likely to become full-time meditators, Davidson's results are still extremely exciting, because they suggest the power of intentional, sustained mental exercise to redesign our neural circuitry.

Inflammation

We know that low-grade inflammation increases as we age, due to an increase in several types of cells of the immune system that secrete multiple troublesome molecules called pro-inflammatory cytokines. These are thought to be a risk factor in a range of age-related diseases, such as hypertension, diabetes, arteriosclerosis, and cancer. While mindfulness meditation cannot cure any known illness, it *can* decrease pro-inflammatory cytokines. The more you practice mindfulness, studies show, the lower your level of pro-inflammatory cytokines, even when you're not meditating.[26]

Increased Telomerase Activity and Telomere Length

You'll recall that telomeres are the little caps on the ends of DNA strands that shorten every time a cell divides. When they get too short, the cell dies. Free radicals, or unstable molecules, can also damage cellular structure. Elizabeth Blackburn won the Nobel Prize for her discovery that the enzyme telomerase helps repair accumulated DNA damage and extend shortened telomeres.

The good news, studies show, is that meditation seems to increase telomerase activity and telomere length,[27] thereby protecting against cellular aging. In an important study, psychologist Elissa Epel and collaborators at UCSF found that meditation boosts telomerase activity by reducing *cognitive stress*.[28] Neuroscientist Clifford Saron's Shamata Project research also found that telomerase activity was 33 percent higher in the meditators who took part in the three-month retreat than in controls.[29] It's also likely that a number of these meditation-influenced factors are *combining* to keep our brains younger. Increasing telomerase activity, decreasing pro-inflammatory cytokines, and lowering the effects of chronic stress may be acting together to reduce normal age-related decline.

Lessening of "Attentional Blink"

Another part of us that tends to worsen with age is the fascinating "attentional blink," which refers to a gap in attention, a fraction of a second of temporary blindness following a period of paying attention.[30] The "blink" is measured by showing people a rapid string of letters interspersed with occasional numbers and asking them to report what numbers they saw. If two numbers are presented in quick succession (within a half-second of the first), most people tend to miss the second number. Those who see more numbers have shorter blinks.

Until recently, scientists assumed the "blink" was unchangeable, a hard-wired aspect of the central nervous system. But then Davidson's group measured the attentional blink in meditators before and after a ten-day Insight Meditation retreat and found a whopping 20 percent reduction in attentional blink, because, they hypothesized, there was less of a response to the first stimulus. In other words, with mindfulness training, people could just "notice" the first stimulus and move on.[31]

As we get older, the attentional blink becomes more frequent and creates longer gaps in our ability to scan our surroundings, which means older people can sometimes miss important information, like quick eye movements signaling a subtle change in another's emotions. Critical things can also happen in that half-second blink that can even affect our safety. A deer might leap into the road; the car in front of you might slam on its brakes.

Wondering whether meditation training might offset the blink's worsening with age, German researchers from the Max Planck Institute for Brain Research[32] found that older meditators who practiced "open monitoring" meditation reversed the usual escalation of attentional blinks with aging, even doing better than another younger group. Open monitoring—that is, having no specific attentional focus in the body—seems to lessen the speed with which the focus of attention is engaged or disengaged. In fact, a Dutch group of scientists found that they could shorten the attentional blink with just seventeen minutes of mindfulness training.[33] It appears that mindfulness enlarges our aperture of attention.

What About Dementia?

How effective are meditation-oriented practices for preventing or slowing age-related dementia? First off, we now know that dementia is *not* an inescapable part of aging. The influential medical journal *The Lancet* recently did a whole issue on the question, and its expert panel concluded: "Dementia is by no means an inevitable consequence of reaching retirement age, or even of entering the ninth decade. . . . *One third of dementia cases may be preventable*."[34] A special recent issue of the *Journal of Alzheimer's Disease* likewise concluded that "aging without dementia is achievable."[35]

All these dementia experts agree on what you can do to preserve your brain health until late in life: take care of your general health through physical activity, a healthy diet, and no smoking; maintain your vascular health by controlling blood pressure, cholesterol, and diabetes; and develop what's called "cognitive reserve" through education, particularly childhood education, social engagement, and mental activities. It's also noteworthy that the incidence of dementia has declined in Europe and North America over the past few decades, providing further evidence that a focus on a healthy lifestyle can lower the risk of dementia in later life.

A deep understanding of dementia is complicated, however, because the various forms seem to arise from many different brain abnormalities and because, despite billions of dollars spent on research, we still do not know what causes, for example, Alzheimer's disease. It has been found that nearly half of centenarians with dementia did not have sufficient brain pathology to explain their cognitive symptoms, while intermediate-to-high Alzheimer's pathology (like tangles and plaques) is present in around one-third of very old people without dementia or cognitive impairment.[36] This again suggests that certain compensatory mechanisms, like cognitive reserve or cognitive resilience, may play a role in helping people in extreme old age escape dementia syndromes.

What about mind-body therapies such as yoga and meditation? These practices are increasingly popular in programs for prevention or treatment of dementia. How effective are they? Yoga and meditation, research shows, can improve symptoms of mild cognitive impairment in older people, and a few studies report these practices helping with severe dementias, like Alzheimer's. But there is no solid evidence that meditative practices can alter the specific pathology underlying Alzheimer's disease or other severe dementias, and most experts conclude that they can appear to improve dementia by boosting health in general.[37]

While I was writing this chapter, I had an unexpected, personal experience of the power of meditation. I was on a walk with a friend when she went into atrial fibrillation (Afib), an irregular heart rhythm that occurs in many older people, that left her feeling weak and light-headed. She began trying different things, like slow breathing, to try to restore her normal heart rhythm. On a hunch, I asked her if she could do an experiment and put her hand on her heart, focus her attention on her heart sensations, and send herself "metta" in a deeply loving way. After only about fifteen seconds, she suddenly stopped, felt her pulse, and said, "I can't believe it! I'm out of Afib!" I offer this experience only as a remarkable personal observation; I don't want to suggest that using metta to stop Afib has been medically proven. Even so, we can safely conclude from all the research that contemplative body practices are highly beneficial for the general brain health and well-being of older people. Now, let's look more closely at other meditative practices like breathing, yoga, chanting, and tai chi, and consider ways they may be uniquely helpful for different kinds of people.

Breathing

Breathing is a crucially important part of any contemplative practice, be it meditation, yoga, tai chi, or other forms. Breath work itself is also an ancient and powerful practice. I want to highlight it here because, while we all take some 25,000 breaths a day, most of us don't do it correctly and don't understand the impact that breathing has on our health and well-being. Even our doctors don't keep tabs on our respiratory health.

In his rollicking, best-selling recent book *Breath: The New Science of a Lost Art*, journalist James Nestor doesn't mince words.[38] He reports that scientists from diverse fields who study breathing estimate that 90 percent of us are breathing incorrectly, causing or aggravating nasal obstructions and many chronic diseases like high blood pressure, asthma, immune disorders, and, of course, anxiety. Around half of us are breathing through our mouths rather than our noses, which is terribly destructive to our health, and women and children are suffering the most. We're also breathing too fast, taking about 3.3 seconds to inhale and exhale, when we should be breathing more slowly and gently, taking air in slowly from pelvis to collarbone and expelling more of it by moving our diaphragms in and out.

Panic disorders, research shows, are caused by rapid, shallow breathing—that is, breathing too much and lowering carbon dioxide to unhealthy levels. In one study, a group of panic sufferers were successfully taught to breathe less and more slowly, increasing their carbon dioxide and reversing the shortness of breath and intolerable feelings of suffocation.[39] So, if you feel a panic attack coming on, it is not helpful to "take a deep breath." Holding your breath is much more effective.

My sixty-three-year-old patient Ruth came into treatment complaining of unbearable anxiety, which manifested in intense neck pain and constant worry about work deadlines. She also had trouble getting to bed on time or giving herself time to eat lunch. For months, we discussed her imperious and dismissive boss and her difficult husband, and, during this time, she was able to make some important life changes. Her anxiety, however, remained much the same. Then I began to notice that Ruth would very often hold her breath for ten seconds or more, and, when I shared my observations, it became clear to both of us that this was agitating both her body and mind. I taught her how to breathe in through her nose from her belly and to exhale slowly and completely, and, after some months, she could finally sometimes do this on her own. Ruth also became more and more aware of her incessant feeling that she was "never ever doing enough" and should always be doing more. She began to realize that, in her frantic need to please others, she could not even allow herself time to breathe fully! Because of this, her body was out of whack. For Ruth, learning how to change an important bodily pattern, her breath, was a crucial first step in learning to value, respect, and take care of her body and herself.

Studies show the most calming and efficient breathing rhythm is 5.5-second inhalations followed by 5.5-second exhalations, which works out almost exactly to 5.5 breaths a minute. Our society considers twelve to twenty breaths a minute normal. Of course, this new knowledge has already been monetized into apps, masks, and mouthpieces that help you inhale and exhale every 5.5 seconds. But you don't need the apps; you just need your nose. If you just breath through your nose more slowly, your nasal tissue (which is erectile tissue!) will take care of the rest. It is naturally flexing constantly, Nestor writes, adjusting the flow of air to suit the current needs of your body and brain.

Breathing well can turn on the vast body network called the autonomic nervous system, which works "automatically" to control inner functions, explains neuroscientist and psychiatrist Stephen Porges.[40] When you breathe slowly through your nose, from your abdomen, and exhale slowly, you are opening up communication along the vagal nerve network, stimulating the parasympathetic wing of your autonomic nervous system, which releases hormones that relax the mind and prompt your organs to rest and digest. Many of the nerves connecting to the para-sympathetic system are located in the lower lobes of your lungs, which is one reason long and slow breaths are so relaxing. You can trigger this calming neurological response at will and at any time or place simply by focusing on your belly while taking long, slow breaths through your nose. Isn't it ironic that so many women learned Lamaze breathing only to promptly forget it after childbirth?

It turns out that much of the autonomic nervous system, which was supposed to be beyond our control, is not. Nestor tracked down people around the world to study the hidden science behind ancient breathing practices like pranayama, sudarshan kriya, and tummo, many of which have recently been repurposed for twenty-first-century life. There had been reports since the early 1900s of Buddhist monks using a heavy-breathing technique called tummo and melting circles in the snow around their bare bodies. A Harvard researcher named Herbert Benson decided to test this and hooked up three monks to sensors as they practiced tummo breath-ing, and he found that their body temperatures did, in fact, rise by as much as seventeen degrees and remain there.[41] More recently, Dutch phenom-enon Wim Hof ran a half-marathon through the snow above the Arctic Circle shirtless and barefooted, as well as a full marathon in the Namib Desert in temperatures reaching 104 degrees, without ever sipping a drop of water. He also had himself injected with *E. coli* and did not get sick. His "method," detailed in his popular book,[42] includes his own version of a heavy-breathing practice, cold exposure, and meditative techniques. Researchers were astounded when a group of people trained in the method were also able to fight off an *E. coli* injection without getting sick. The Wim Hof breathing method is also highly adaptable and has been incorporated into a wellness training program for older people.

Obviously, my aim is not to encourage you to undertake wild, crazy, and dangerous feats. I offer these extreme examples as more evidence of how malleable our bodies can be with targeted training, and how they can lose function without training. *This is so important for us as we age.* Without exercise, our lungs will lose 12 percent of their capacity from age thirty to fifty (with women faring worse than men), and by the time we reach eighty we'll be able to take in 30 percent less air than we did in our twenties. Researchers at the University of Buffalo studied more than a thousand subjects over three decades to find out if lung size really did correlate to longevity, as the famous Framingham study from the 1980s had suggested. They found that, yes, larger lungs led to longer lives.[43] The smaller and less efficient their lungs became, the earlier the subjects got sick and died. Luckily, any regular practice that stretches the lungs can retain or increase lung capacity. Even moderate exercise like walking or cycling has been shown to boost lung size by up to 15 percent.

There are dozens of breathing techniques, which either heat up or cool the body and/or expand the lungs. I'll share three that I find particularly useful.

Resonant (Coherent) Breathing

Here, in more detail, is the calming practice Nestor recommends to shift the heart, lungs, and circulation into a state of coherence, in which the systems of the body are working at peak efficiency. According to many breathing experts, there is no more essential technique, and none more basic.

- Sit up straight, relax the shoulders and belly, and exhale.

- Inhale softly for 5.5 seconds, expanding the belly as air fills the bottom of the lungs.

- Without pausing, exhale softly for 5.5 seconds, bringing the belly in as the lungs empty. Each breath should feel like a circle.

- Repeat at least ten times, more if possible.

4-7-8 Breathing

This technique, which comes from Andrew Weil, is deeply relaxing and can help you fall asleep.

- Take a breath in, then exhale through your mouth with a *whoosh* sound.

- Close your mouth and inhale quietly through your nose to a mental count of four.

- Hold for a count of seven.

- Exhale completely through your mouth with a whoosh, to the count of eight.

- Repeat this cycle for at least four breaths.

Weil's instructional video is available online. But don't expect this one to be easy when you first try it. You may have to work your way into this technique.

Yawning

I personally find that the simple, natural act of yawning is the fastest way to transform an uptight body into a more relaxed, aware one. To trigger a transformative yawn, first inhale slowly and deeply, then exhale very slowly, making a continuous "ssssssss" sound through your mouth. As you continue to exhale, you may be able to sense the muscles of your jaw, neck, and mouth "wanting" to yawn. Allow these sensations to increase into a series of inhalations that trigger a great big yawn. What pleasure! The enjoyment you feel comes from stimulating the parasympathetic nervous system, which increases relaxation and feelings of well-being.

Yoga

The modern yoga craze, where millions of (mostly) women flock to group classes at yoga studios, is a far cry from the way Asian yogis have practiced for thousands of years and continue to practice today.[44] Traditionally, the yogi (practitioner) would meet with his guru (teacher) in a remote location and would engage in lengthy yoga poses (asanas) and pranayama breathing in order to evoke meditative states. The modern yoga format, with its sets of seated and standing poses and its "yoga flow," was actually lifted from European exercise routines. There are now some 21 million practitioners in the United States, and 250 million worldwide, mostly white, educated, higher-earning women.

The earliest yoga was, in fact, a science of holding still and building *prana* through breathing. The oldest documented artifact of a yogic posture, found in the 1920s in the Indus Valley, is of a man sitting erect with his hands on his knees. Yoga was one of hundreds of ways that the ancients devised to open up channels in the body that contained the "life force" or "vital energy." The most powerful technique was to inhale prana, to *breathe*, and the first compilation of yoga techniques, *Yoga Sutras of Patanjali*, describes various breathing practices, including some I described earlier.

Yoga is a kind of moving meditation. In fact, in meditation retreats, yoga is more and more often included as an important daily part of the retreat. Because it draws your attention inward and encourages you to pay careful and continuous attention to your body sensations, it is yet another way to cultivate interoceptive awareness, while also strengthening and stretching the muscles. In fact, yoga is more and more frequently called "yoga therapy." Almost three-quarters of practitioners say they use yoga for general well-being and disease prevention. People who attend therapeutic yoga classes come most often for back/neck pain (77 percent), joint pain/stiffness (67 percent), and anxiety (77 percent).[45]

My interviewee and old friend Lily, now sixty-three, has been faithfully practicing yoga for thirty years. I asked her what she'd learned over all those years:

> Well, I'd always had a kind of macho approach to athletic things, and that's what yoga was about when I started. It was about "working out" and trying to push my body into harder and harder poses. I still remember this day when I confidently moved to the wall and into a handstand for the first time and felt very proud. Then my teacher came over and gently said, "Lily, that's not bad, but you will hurt yourself." She had me pull my elbow in, so it was aligned with my shoulder, which made the pose much safer. That experience really shifted things for me. I realized how much I could be pulled into being competitive and ego-driven and that this practice was different—that yoga was ultimately about working with my body with gentleness and attunement.
>
> I think my practice also really changed when I became pregnant at age thirty-eight, which is late to get pregnant. Giving birth deepened my sense of really appreciating my body and all

it could do and my need to keep it healthy. I realized I not only needed to nurture my kids but to nurture myself. Yoga gave me a place to go to practice and nurture myself, which enabled me to be a better mother. I found it deeply, emotionally grounding. Even if my kids were balking about my leaving, I went to yoga! Yoga was a commitment to myself.

Now as an older woman, I still recognize a certain competitiveness in me, like when I think, "At sixty-three, I can still do these things younger people can't do," but I don't usually think that way these days. Yoga has taught me to work with my body's limitations, to work with my body as it is now. Yoga feels more like a spiritual practice than a sport. One of the most powerful yoga experiences I've had is when I had to relearn how to do the backbend, which I'd done so easily as a kid. At this point, I had these limitations in my body . . . and also my fear. So, I had to visualize doing the backbend without really doing it for, maybe, four years, as I worked with my fear and my physical limitations. It felt so good when I finally did it! I realize now that yoga is about letting yourself work with the building blocks of who you are, rather than this Western thing of pushing yourself to be who you think you should be. The whole process is so heart-opening.

Yoga is extremely good for us as we age, since it puts less strain on the body than traditional sports, as well as focusing us inward. But, as Lily warned us, we have to do yoga carefully and safely with a highly trained teacher we trust. There has been some concern recently about yoga injuries, but the data on yoga injuries shows that most are the result of the more athletic and adventurous poses like the hand-, shoulder-, and headstands, most involving overbending or overextending the spine. In fact, yoga researchers report that yoga does not produce more injuries than nonyoga exercise.[46]

There's a type or level of yoga for everyone; a dozen or more common varieties range from more traditional forms like Hatha, Iyengar, and Ashtanga to gentler types like Yin yoga or restorative yoga, to more athletic types like Power Yoga or Bikram ("hot") or Vinyasa ("flow"), to Kundalini, which includes chanting and singing, to aerial yoga, in which you are suspended from a strong, silky hammock hanging from the ceiling. Here's my Yin yoga teacher:

> As you sit on your mat, allow your breath to become more conscious, more full, and deep. There's no right or wrong here. From your sitting posture, slowly lower your back to the mat, vertebra by vertebra, slowly, slowly. If you feel any discomfort at all in your lower back, slightly raise your knees. Now gently raise your right arm and place your right hand on your left shoulder, as you are able.... Do not strain.... Let your own body be your guide.

My teacher is not only trying to prevent injury. She is also focusing my attention inward and encouraging me to deeply and meticulously attend to my body sensations and comfort.

While the scientific research specifically on yoga is not as voluminous as for meditation, it is still massive, with over a thousand studies published since the 1970s, and numbers soaring in the past few years. Yoga's wonderful benefits are fundamentally the same as those of meditation—increased interoceptive awareness and all that follows from that, like better emotion regulation, sharpened attention, increased compassion, decreased anxiety and depression, and more reliable parasympathetic activation.

In addition to offering these more general benefits of meditation, yoga, because of its movement component, increases flexibility, muscle strength and tone, and balance. It also appears to hold promise for certain pain syndromes like migraine, lower-back pain, and fibromyalgia.[47] Yoga and other movement practices are also particularly effective for people with anxiety and panic, in part because it is so deeply relaxing and, also, because it can often be tolerated better than meditation by highly anxious people who may find it unendurable to sit with their anxious and negative thoughts.

I think of my patient Carol, age sixty-eight, who has suffered from crippling anxiety, self-doubt, and perfectionism all her life. Some years ago, I suggested she look into meditation and/or yoga, and I was surprised when she immediately decided to try meditation. She tried it repeatedly but always ended up depressed because she couldn't bear watching her anxious, ruminative, self-hating thoughts. She also always felt she wasn't doing it "right," because her mind wandered, as everyone's does. Meditation made her feel worse about herself. So then, with lots of trepidation, Carol decided to try yoga. It felt like a big stretch, because she had always felt painfully shy in groups. She finally got herself to a class, and then, that very same week, she went to another and another, until she found a teacher she really liked. When she next came to see me, she said very decisively, "I'm going to do this!" Soon she was going to yoga three, sometimes four, times a week, and she reported feeling much more relaxed and less self-hating. Yoga fit Carol like a key in a lock—it opened her up!

Chanting

Many forms of meditation and yoga also include *sound*. Chanting mantras and singing powerfully focus attention on the body and build interoceptive awareness. In these practices, you can actually *feel* the sound vibrations inside your body. What a wonderful feeling! Whether you are vocalizing the sound of "om" or a special mantra, or chanting ancient Buddhist, Jewish, Christian, Muslim, or Hindu prayers, the rhythmic breathing and simple repetition tethers you to the present moment, slowing your breathing and brain activity and relaxing your body by stimulating your vagus nerve and parasympathetic nervous system. Chanting also calms the fight/flight reaction of the amygdala, while, at the same time, activating the "higher" areas of the brain responsible for empathy and compassion.

These benefits are dramatically increased when you chant with a group, synchronizing your breathing and biorhythms with those around you. Singer Heather Houston offers lovely classes and retreats on "The Art of Mindful Singing," which include mantras, chants, and other "vocal meditation" to promote greater body health and well-being.[48] You can also check local listings for *kirtan* or other singing groups or choirs in your community.

Tai Chi

Another practice that explicitly cultivates interoceptive awareness is tai chi, along with its close relative, qigong. Tai chi is an ancient Chinese martial art that integrates a series of weight shifting, body rotations, and semi-squat exercises with deep-breathing techniques. Its slow, flowing body movements require the coordination of head, eyes, arms, torso, pelvis, and legs, which promotes flexibility, strengthening, and stress relief.

While tai chi is wonderful for all ages, it is highly recommended for older adults because it can be gentle and performed without aggravating existing impairments and doesn't require getting down on the floor. It is incredibly safe: its circular movements keep muscles relaxed with minimal strain on bones and joints. Tai chi may be easily adapted for every age and fitness level. Qigong, another form of flowing, standing movement with multiple benefits, is an alternative practice, which many people prefer because it's easier to learn. Its name reveals its close connection to breathing: *Qi* means "breath," and gong means "work." *Breath work.*

Tai chi, the research shows, significantly increases bodily awareness in older adults.[49] Older people who practice tai chi are less likely to fall than nonpractitioners, because they have learned to more fully and accurately feel the sensation of their feet on the ground and because they are more present and less preoccupied. Tai chi also brings significant brain benefits, including increases in brain volume, delayed dementia, and improvements on tests of memory and thinking.[50] Because tai chi and qigong, like yoga, cultivate interoceptive awareness, they strengthen our sense of well-being, agency, and self-awareness.

When I was in China some years ago, I not only saw older people doing tai chi and qigong and other martial arts in the public parks but also saw them walking barefooted back and forth over stone paths during the morning hours. What was going on? I did some research and found out that Chinese elders have, since ancient times, been walking or dancing or exercising on stone paths as a way of maintaining mobility and staying young. Researchers at the Oregon Research Institute studied this practice and found that people over age sixty who walked on a specially designed mat to simulate cobblestones for a half-hour a day over four months significantly lowered their blood pressure and improved their balance and mobility, compared to a control group who walked on an even surface.[51] The researchers hypothesized that walking on cobblestones forces you to continuously adjust your balance, thereby strengthening your vestibular system, and it also likely stimulates reflexology and acupressure points on the soles of the feet. Maybe this is why Chinese people appear to remain so animated and healthy into old age.

Other Mindfulness-Oriented Healing Methods

Feldenkrais, the Alexander Method, Pilates, Focusing, Rosen Method bodywork, Hakomi, Somatic Experiencing, Acceptance and Commitment Therapy, and Dialectical-Behavioral Therapy all focus to some extent on mindfulness or interoceptive practices. If you are interested, I suggest you try different ones, because people respond so differently to different techniques—recall Carol, who responded negatively to meditation but so enthusiastically to yoga. Do you want a body therapy, like the Rosen Method, in which you can also explore psychological issues through releasing body constriction? Or do you particularly want to improve body posture with the Alexander Method? We are lucky to be at this moment in history when we have so many choices about how to guide our bodies through the unpredictable terrain of our later years.

As I stated in chapter 3, I believe that all psychotherapies at their best involve the ongoing somatic awareness of the patient as well as the therapist. As a psychotherapist myself, I often try to elicit those regions of the patient's brain that monitor and represent the internal state of the body with questions like, "What do you notice in your body right now?" followed by questions like, "What happens when you focus in on that sensation?" Psychotherapy can be surprisingly useful in reinstating *body* development, as well as emotional development, from the point where it may have gotten derailed earlier in life.

Exercise

By no means do I want to denigrate regular exercise—it's just not a focus of this book. I myself love to walk, swim, cycle, and lift weights. When we work out our bodies, we're not only getting "fit," we're learning more about how our body operates and what it needs to work best. We now know that exercise, particularly the aerobic variety, triggers the release of special chemicals associated with growth that combat those associated with the decline of aging. According to one best-selling exercise book,[52] our brain can only respond to what the body is telling it. If our body is active, our brain thinks, "Ah, she's still a contender, let's keep pumping out chemicals that help her keep on growing and thriving." However, if we are not active, our brain thinks, "Ah, she must be weak and dying" and triggers chemicals that slowly weed us out of the population.

Findings from a recent, huge meta-study reveal that the sweet spot for exercise is about thirty-five minutes a day of brisk walking or other moderate activities. This amount led to the greatest statistical improvement in life span, no matter how many hours one spent sitting.[53] Mounting research shows that many problems associated with aging—like weakness, sore joints, balance issues, poor posture, slowness, and fatigue—can be delayed until almost the end of life by exercising, unless of course we develop serious dysfunction. Moderately physically active women also have lower levels of cancer, heart attack, and stroke, greater longevity, and sharper minds.

"Forest Bathing"

What the Japanese call "forest bathing" (*shinrin-yoku*), now something of an international fad, is simply being in the presence of trees in a relaxed, open, and unhurried way. Most of us already know how good it feels to immerse ourselves in the scents, sounds, and transcendent visual beauty of the forest. It eases stress, rejuvenates, brings us into the present, and increases well-being.

We know, and yet we forget. So, it's good to have mounting scientific evidence that "forest bathing" transforms the health of our bodies as well as our minds. Studies by researchers, including Qing Li[54] in Japan, Dacher Keltner in Berkeley, and hundreds of others around, the world reveal that immersion in nature can lower heart rate and blood pressure, reduce cortisol, and boost immune function through increasing natural killer (NK) cell activity and anticancer proteins. Needless to say, our older bodies can particularly benefit.

Creative Pursuits

It's also crucial, as we age, to stay curious, and keep on learning and finding creative outlets. Your mind stays young by staying active, seeking out new information, entertaining new ideas, wandering into new territory. The creative arts, in particular, exercise and stretch the brain, because each new song, poem, or dance requires looking at things differently, opening up new areas of the brain and creating novel connections between different brain areas. Creative activities that have a *physical* component, like music, painting, sculpture, quilting, pottery, and woodworking, appear to be particularly helpful in combating dementia.[55]

Biofeedback and Neurofeedback

In the most advanced forms of biofeedback, people can see a display of their own brain activity and, using real-time fMRI, actively experiment with making body/brain changes to increase internal awareness. Or they can watch animated representations of brain activity. In one neurofeedback study with chronic pain patients,[56] investigators at Stanford Medical Center presented a computer-animated flickering flame that represented their pain. The patients learned to use neurofeedback to lower the flame, thereby decreasing their pain. Neurofeedback is also being used successfully to treat anxiety and depression.

Sense It—Fix It!

Another exciting part of building body awareness is that you become more aware of parts of your body that aren't working properly and, sometimes, how to fix them. In fact, you can become aware of aspects of your body that have *never* worked right, and you can even repair some of those! I offer two of my own examples.

As I mentioned at the very beginning of this book, I often walk on a lovely, tree-lined fire trail near my home. Particularly if I'm alone, I allow myself to focus on the sensations of my body walking and breathing, the songs of the birds, the rustling of the leaves, the squirrels breaking small branches in the trees, and the scent of pine needles warmed by the sun. I'd had a problem with my right knee since I stepped up on a rock while carrying a heavy pack when backpacking in my twenties. I now knew that I needed to keep the muscles around the knee strong to hold it in place, and I'd gotten good orthotics that really helped, but that knee would still sometimes give me trouble. One day, when I was walking in a particularly mindful way, I realized I was slightly "supinating," walking on the outside of my right foot, and then and there I decided to make a conscious effort to walk on the whole foot—rolling, as recommended, from the heel through the ball of the foot and off the big toe. I practiced this for some weeks until it started feeling natural, correcting myself when I forgot and started pronating again. Well, lo and behold, that knee pain, which had been with me at that point for over forty years, completely went away and never returned! I had received physical therapy for the knee pain two different times, but because the therapists had addressed only the knee itself and not the misalignment caused by the supination, the knee pain never completely resolved. Of course, you can argue that another physical therapist, chiropractor, or body worker might have fixed the problem, and I would agree with you; sometimes you need to consult multiple experts for stubborn problems, and I'm all for getting the help you need. My point here, though, is how much you can do for *yourself* when you are deeply and continuously aware of your body and how it feels as it moves in space. No one knows better than *you* how you feel—a truism, yes, but often not heeded.

Now, the plot thickens and does include a physical therapist. I had sprained my right foot a few months previously and finally decided to consult a highly respected PT. He had numerous ideas about how to work on my foot/ankle through manual therapy as well as lots of strengthening and balance exercises. At one point I remarked that I had "flat feet," and he said "No, you don't, you have high arches; it's just that they've collapsed." This was big news to me! In the enlightened 1950s of my childhood, I had "wedges" added to the soles of my saddle shoes to raise my arches, and I was also instructed to "walk on the outsides of my feet," which I dutifully continued to do for the next sixty-eight years. This same "progressive" shoe store I was taken to as a kid also had an X-ray machine, which allowed you to see your foot inside the shoe, and we kids spent as much time as we could in that machine, happily irradiating our feet.

My physical therapist then proceeded without fanfare to teach me how to actually build arches! First, he had me activate my glutes, abs, and pelvic floor, then tighten (pull up on) the muscles of my inner foot. He also suggested a slight outward rotation of my right hip, which allowed a bone in my right foot to move into place, allowing an arch to naturally appear! Unbelievable! After a few months of these foot exercises, I had respectable arches for the first time in my life. Who knew? Certainly not any of my doctors throughout my life. It sure would have helped to have possessed those arches in my childhood, when I wore toe shoes for ballet, or later, when I wanted to dress up in strappy little sandals.

My main point is this: don't accept your physical limitations just because they've been with you forever or for a very long time. Don't assume there's nothing you can do about them. Don't assume you have to feel this way forever. We have a wide range of highly trained practitioners, like physical therapists, chiropractors, massage therapists, and all the mindfulness-oriented practitioners I mentioned earlier, who can work miracles with our bodies. We now know that we have the power to transform our own bodies and brains through our breath, movement, and attention. Our bodies turn out to be so much more capable of change than we ever imagined. I urge you to explore all the opportunities our amazingly resourceful, health-conscious culture has to offer. Don't give up.

Diet

Knowing how to eat also requires body awareness. You cannot feel your internal body sensations if there is too much interference from too much sugar, saturated fat, caffeine, alcohol, and so on. Your body cannot operate optimally without the right nutrients. When you agitate or scramble or dampen your body's internal signals by eating the wrong foods, you are interfering with your brain's ability to respond to your internal world of sensation/emotion and to the external world around you; and, as you have learned, you are not as effective in maintaining your homeostasis. You are less regulated. It's not just a cute saying that "you are what you eat."

I still love Michael Pollan's seven-word diet recommendation from a few years ago[57]: "Eat food. Not too much. Mostly plants." Current US government dietary guidelines say basically the same thing. They recommend:

- A variety of vegetables—dark green, red, and orange, legumes (beans and peas), starchy and otherwise.

- Fruits, especially whole fruits.

- Grains, at least half of which are whole grains.

- Fat-free or low-fat dairy, including milk, yogurt, cheese, and/or fortified soy beverages.

- Limited saturated fats.

- Limited red meat and processed meats.

- Limited sugar—10 percent of calories.

- Limited salt—less than 2,300 milligrams daily.

Many nutrition scientists, like those from the Buck Foundation for Aging in Marin County, California, suggest that a daily twelve-hour "fast" (i.e., not eating anything for twelve hours out of every twenty-four-hour period, which many of us can do quite easily overnight) can increase life span as well as health.

As mentioned in chapter 4, it is our gut microbiome that analyzes the food we eat and figures out how to optimally digest or reject it. However, as we age, the *diversity* and resilience of the microbes living in our gut decreases, which can weaken our immune system, making us somewhat more vulnerable to various digestive disorders and irritable bowel syndrome, as well as anxiety, depression, fatigue, and certain degenerative disorders of the aging brain, like Alzheimer's or Parkinson's disease. So, it's particularly important as we get older to make sure our aging gut gets the food and care it needs to remain healthy and strong. Brain-gut expert Emeran Mayer suggests how we can tune up our microbiome and maintain our physical and mental health with a few simple changes to our diet and lifestyle[58]:

- Maximize gut microbial diversity by regularly eating naturally fermented foods that contain "good" live bacteria and yeasts ("probiotics")—like yogurt, sauerkraut, miso, kimchi, or kombucha—or taking probiotic supplements found in pharmacies.

- Reduce inflammation in your gut microbiome by:
    - Cutting down on animal fat (including cheese) in your diet.
    - Avoiding mass-produced, processed food (which can contain dangerous additives like artificial sweeteners or emulsifiers) and selecting organically grown food.
    - Eating smaller servings at meals.
    - Reducing stress and practicing mindfulness.
    - Not eating when you are stressed, angry, or sad.
    - Enjoying the pleasure and social aspects of food.
    - Listening to your gut feelings.

What about the dozens of popular diets like Keto, Paleo, and Whole30? Diets like these attract so much hype and so much conflicting science that, I think, you just have to find your own way. First, talk with a very trusted health-care provider who knows your particular physical health strengths and challenges, and then, if you want to try a special diet, proceed carefully and slowly, trying to be aware of its effects on your body at each step of the way. To determine whether a food or diet is truly good for you, use your growing body awareness to deeply tune into your entire body and how every part of it is reacting to the new regime. You must weigh the opinions of your health experts with your own internal understanding of your body, which you have gained over a lifetime. For example, some people "know" that chocolate gives them a blood sugar spike that leads to a headache and a general feeling of malaise but still can't really acknowledge what they know. You must be honest with yourself about what you already know and what you are continually learning about your body.

Sleep

We are finally recognizing that adequate sleep is absolutely essential for our health and well-being, after underestimating its importance for too long. Getting enough sleep—seven to eight hours a night—is as crucial as exercise and diet in preserving brain/body function. Neuropsychologist

Matthew Walker's definitive book *Why We Sleep* has been a major catalyst in waking us up to the power of sleep. It is during sleep that we consolidate memories, heal tissue, boost our immune system, control our hormonal cycles, and "rinse" our brains of toxic waste. Sleep keeps us attentive, creative, quick thinking, and happier.

Scientists estimate that two-thirds of us living in the modern developed world are chronically sleep deprived, which puts us at higher risk for dementia, depression, mood disorders, memory problems, heart disease, high blood pressure, weight gain and obesity, fall-related injuries, cancer, and increased negative thinking. Note that all of these health challenges show up frequently in older people.

What is probably most familiar to those of us with sleep deprivation, besides fatigue, is its effect on *memory*. We all know the experience of "brain fog," which comes over us after a bad night or two, or more, of sleep. Without proper sleep, research shows, memories cannot be consolidated and organized and filed away for future recall.[59] It's not surprising, but still disturbing, therefore, that older adults with poor sleep have higher rates of cognitive decline and are more likely to get Alzheimer's disease.[60]

Lack of sleep also adversely affects hunger, appetite, and body image. One study shows that people who slept just four hours a night for two consecutive nights experienced a 24 percent increase in hunger and gravitated toward high-calorie treats, salty snacks, and starchy foods, which led to weight gain.[61]

As we age, our sleep cycles change naturally in certain ways. We have more trouble getting to sleep and staying asleep, and we tend to go to bed earlier and wake up earlier, but we continue to need just as much sleep as when we were younger. Poor sleep is not inevitable or normal. We do need to watch our "sleep hygiene," however, including:

- Stick to a schedule by going to bed and getting up at the same time every day, including weekends and holidays. Going to bed before midnight and waking up with early morning light is ideal to preserve natural sleep cycles.

- Avoid caffeine after lunch and go easy on alcohol, since both disrupt normal sleep cycles.

- Beware of side effects of medications: for example, medications for headaches and colds can contain stimulants, and anti-anxiety meds can disrupt restorative slow-wave sleep.

- Keep your bedroom cool, quiet, and dark. Banish electronics, which contain blue wavelengths that suppress melatonin, the hormone needed for sleep.

- Give yourself at least thirty minutes to "wind down" and relax before going to bed—perhaps with the help of a mindful body scan or calming breathing practice.

Sensual Enjoyment

When you enhance your interoceptive abilities, studies show, you can also appreciate *pleasant sensations* more. You're more able to really *enjoy* your body. For example, when you eat mindfully, you bring more attention to the pleasure of seeing, smelling, tasting, and eating foods. I cannot tell you how intensely pleasurable meals become when you are on a meditation retreat and living more in your body with few distractions. Flavors pop and expand in unfamiliar ways, and you want your mealtimes to last forever!

Those of us who are not able to enter into such pleasurable sensory states and appreciate positive sensations can have trouble regulating ourselves. For example, studies show, people whose brains' reward regions respond less to the pleasures of food are more likely to gain unwanted weight.[62] Because they can't really satisfy their food cravings, they "chase the flavor" and continue eating. What helps? You guessed it—mindfulness training to increase internal sensory awareness.

So, elevate your senses! And see what happens. Music crashes over you in waves. Natural landscapes glow with psychedelic intensity. Massage, cuddling, and hot baths plunge you into delicious stupor. Sex becomes rapture. I think of the wonderful writer and feminist Audre Lorde, who many years ago wrote about the "uses of the erotic." For her, the erotic goes way beyond sexuality. Entering into *eros*, she says, unleashes "the power of all of our unexpressed and all of our unrecognized feelings."

Chapter 7

Our Aging Bodies,
Our Aging Selves

"I love my body; I feel like my body is my old friend who's stayed with me all these years."

I absolutely love this comment from Edna, age eighty-three, who delivered it during her interview with a little smile. And it was eye-opening for me when nearly all the thirty women I interviewed, who ranged in age from forty-eight to ninety-one, told me that their lives had gotten *better* in many ways as they got older, despite their fears of all the unknowns of aging:

"I feel a lot more freedom to acknowledge how I feel and *move* on it," said Addy, age sixty-three. "I can call the shots."

"I don't care anymore if I'm really thin and totally fit. These things just don't matter so much. I want to go into nature," said Lisa, age seventy-one.

"I feel more related to my body than when I was younger," said Suzanne, age fifty-eight. "My body's less of a thing outside me and more 'me.'"

No one, of course, expressed delight about the wrinkling and the sagging of their flesh, but more than half did say they'd come to some kind of "it is what it is" acceptance, and many even said that they felt "grateful" to their bodies for carrying them this far. It was also striking to me that every single woman I interviewed mentioned feeling less anxious, and almost all reported something in the realm of feeling "more like myself." *Less anxious . . . more like myself.* These are huge changes that profoundly transform our experience of living.

The fact is, much as we dislike the descending of the flesh, it is the aging of the body that sets the stage for and ushers in our ultimate stage of life, a distinct new phase with its own advantages, challenges, and surprising revelations. It is the aging of the body that spurs surprising new psychological development in later life.

What the Body Does for Us

Let's consider some of the things we've learned about the body so far. For starters, we now know that our body is not just a "temple" we live in, or a "vehicle" for carrying us around, or a stand for our computer/brain. Our body *is* us. It is integral not only to our functioning but also to creating our emotional sense of ourselves. Our body is the foundation of our being. How we feel *about* our bodies is not merely a reflection of how beautiful or strong or healthy or competent our bodies are but depends to a large degree on how we feel *in* our bodies, which, in turn, depends on how *aware* we are of our bodies. As you now know, there is a direct physiological link between being able to viscerally sense our bodies and being able to regulate, maintain, and restore our physical and emotional health. We feel happier, more alive, more peaceful, and more grounded when we are embodied. How comfortable we are in our bodies also depends on how *others* have responded to our bodies throughout our lives.

Our ability to register and interpret the profusion of sensory signals from inside our bodies is also crucial to *aging* successfully. Strong interoceptive awareness helps us take good care of our bodies, as well as our psyches, as we get older. Unlike our often-misguided thinking brains, our bodies know what's real for us. Using information from inside and outside our bodies to make predictions, our interoceptive pathways determine what we need to do to maintain our physiological homeostasis, our healthy functioning. As the research on meditation dramatically shows, paying close attention to our body sensations can change us in incredibly important ways—including sharpening our attention, regulating our emotions, lowering inflammation, increasing empathy and compassion, and even increasing our longevity. Neuroplasticity is real. We can change our brains and our bodies at *any* age. Remember, I built arches in my seventy-four-year-old feet!

We've also learned that people with a greater ability to detect internal body sensations have a more accurate and stable body image, as well as greater bodily satisfaction, and stronger body boundaries. Deeper body awareness also helps us resist the brainwashing of our sexist, visual culture. Without a well-developed sense of our body, our body image will not feel real and connected to our full being and will be more of an abstract, and often inaccurate, idea of who we are. For so many reasons, the best brain is an embodied brain.

Brain Aging Unlocks New Capacities

It is also true that certain brain changes that come with aging unlock new kinds of emotional development—changes that have not been acknowledged enough by other writers on aging. I want to focus again on some of the brain functions that change in ways that help us elevate our well-being. We should try to harness the natural strengths of this stage of life, as we do with any other.

First off, you'll remember from chapter 4 that our interoceptive awareness declines as we get older, which means that our bodies are less aroused by and reactive to various internal sensations and emotions. We have fewer negative emotions, particularly anger, and a greater sense of well-being. You'll also recall that, as we age, we're able to take more cognitive control, to change our focus of attention and direct it toward more *positive* goals or memories. Our move toward more positive thinking also stems from the age-related decline of the amygdala, the part of the brain responsible for emotional reactions, particularly negative ones.

But while our internal body signals are weaker, our *perception* and interpretation of them becomes more complex, after many years of trying out different possibilities and learning what works and what doesn't. We can "do more" with our body sensations, as Sahib Khalsa told me. The more experience we have, the better we are at noticing patterns and predicting future outcomes. For example: you feel a little gut wrench when your partner criticizes you, and, in the past, you might have launched a verbal zinger in their direction. But now, having learned from experience that that particular move gets you nowhere, you interpret your gut reaction as a cue to take a breath, look directly at them with eyebrows raised, and say nothing—which is so much more effective. We accumulate a repertoire of strategies over a lifetime. It also helps that abstract reasoning, pattern recognition,[1] and "out-of-the-box" thinking all improve with age, which helps us excel in our area of expertise more than ever before. Artistic creativity can also blossom as we age.[2]

The fact that we are more easily *distracted* as we get older may well be an integral part of these changes. While distractibility is usually considered a negative characteristic, one experiment found that older people, after being distracted, showed much greater ability to solve verbal problems.[3] It appears that heightened distractibility can help us find creative solutions on unusual byways.

The Benefits of Aging

So now, let's look at some of the psychological advantages, or benefits, of getting older, which can arise from these neurophysiological changes as well as the greater experience of age.

Happiness

Certainly, the biggest news about aging is that we are happier, more optimistic, and more emotionally regulated than we were when we were younger! As I've mentioned, research from many quarters confirms that people over the age of sixty-five have the most stable and optimistic outlook of all adults. We older people suffer less from depression, anxiety, and substance abuse. We have fewer negative emotions, and we're better at dealing with hotly charged emotional conflicts and debates. You'll recall that Laura Carstensen labeled this approach a "positivity bias,"[4] which means we older people lean more toward the *positive* in appraising the relationships and events of our lives.

Our greater happiness is graphically and unforgettably presented in what's come to be known as the "U-curve of happiness." According to a three-decade-long University of Chicago study, we are happiest in our younger and older years.[5] Happiness tends to decrease beginning in our late thirties and then begins to increase sharply after age fifty-four, with age eighty-two being the happiness peak! These findings hold true across seventy-two countries, from Albania to Zimbabwe. Another important, recent study of fifteen hundred adults ages twenty-one to one hundred years, led by San Diego aging researcher Dilip Jeste, also found that the older the person, the better his or her mental health tended to be—and that older women's happiness ratings were consistently higher than those of men![6]

Quite remarkable findings, are they not, given the manifold losses and difficulties of aging? Isn't it counterintuitive that we are happier, despite having more aches and pains, less agility, slower mental processes, and so on? Why on earth are older people so happy? Again, it's in large part due to age-related brain/body changes. As our bodies and brains become less reactive and agitated, and our higher-brain control increases, we can more easily direct our attention toward the positive. Then we start to spend more of our available time doing things we *like*, rather than things we should be doing out of obligation or to burnish our image. We make the most of what we have. You bet we're happier!

Perspective

If we turn our gaze back to all the years we have already lived, what do we find? A huge accretion of experience. As our life cycle continues to open out behind us, we have more and more to look back on. We see the endless repetitions of our own behavior patterns and those of humankind-at-large, and it becomes harder and harder not to notice and take stock. We have a greater sense of the whole. We gain "perspective."

As with a novel, it's only at the end that we can see more clearly what it's all been about. As I slowly advance toward my own end, I can almost see my life as a story with well-developed themes, "voice," and characters, a story that I am continuing to write and revise, adding new themes and characters and stumbling upon surprising plot twists, new character development, and unexpected happiness. As the years pile up behind me, the essence of my life—with its unique contours, textures, and hues—comes increasingly into focus, like a photographic image emerging from the developer.

As we get older, our brains become better at "pattern recognition."[7] Recognizing patterns starts at a young age, when we start noticing certain regularities in our world and begin to *generalize*. For example, as little kids, we notice that even though our favorite food comes in many different shapes—corkscrew, tube, bowtie—they all have that same wonderful feel and taste, particularly when topped with spaghetti sauce. And almost all of us, throughout our lives, can meet someone we've never met before and say, "Excuse me, are you by any chance Cynthia's sister (or Cynthia's mother or Cynthia's daughter)?" because our brains are remarkably good at picking up family resemblance, based on abstract generalizations of certain facial features. As we get older and have more perspective, we're more and more able to find patterns where younger people cannot. We're also better at disregarding small details that don't matter, which makes us faster and better at seeing the "big picture."

As we age, we have more and more "ages" inside us.[8] We contain and are constituted by all the ages we have already lived, and with our brain's amazing ability to abstract and synthesize, we experience all these different ages as "me" in a surprisingly embodied way. We experience all our different-aged selves simultaneously within us, with all their different body sensations, feelings, physical dexterities, vulnerabilities, behaviors, preferences, and quirks, and we can feel the synergy of their ongoing negotiations, struggles, and collaborations. I still experience the "giggles" of my ten-year-old self, the wild dancing of my twenty-year-old self, and the deep-hearted maternal concern of my fifty-year-old self. This gives us a tremendous advantage over younger people. No age is a stranger to us. Having ever more ages within us allows us to empathize with and identify with ever more people of all different ages, including their internal ages. The more "ages" we have available, the more analogies and deep streams of connection we can find between ourselves and others.

As we develop greater perspective and gather more memories of what works and what doesn't, we naturally want to pass on what we have learned, to be a link in the chain of knowledge passed down through the generations. Psychoanalyst Erik Erikson called this "generativity," which he defined as "the interest in establishing and guiding the next generation."[9] We become generative not only through parenting or grandparenting but also through myriad forms of altruistic activity and creativity: mentoring, teaching, friendship, taking care of a pet, creating art, or, for me, doing psychotherapy or singing. In being generative, we feel more profoundly connected to other human beings, part of a net of nurturing relationships. Our wider, longer view gives us insight into what matters most in life. We become more able to sustain love for the important people in our lives despite their provocations and shortcomings. We let our sense of self "expand" to include our loved ones, and we actually "carry" our loved ones inside us, in an embodied way.

Our sense of our embodied self can also subjectively "expand" to include the natural world, the planet, or even the universe. Rather than feeling separate and alone, we can experience ourselves, in body and mind, as part of the web of life. Psychoanalyst Heinz Kohut called this "cosmic narcissism," which "transcends the bounds of the individual,"[10] and he believed that it can cushion us in later life from the reality that our own personal lives must come to an end.

A Different Sense of Time

With our widening perspective as we age, our relationship to time also changes. Carstensen points out that we human beings are unique in the animal kingdom in our ability to measure the passage of time against a sort of internal "life-span clock," which keeps track of where we are in the life cycle.[11] When we are young, time seems expansive, and we are pulled to acquire knowledge, seek novel experiences, and engage ourselves in a large network of friends and workmates. As we age, we sense the clock winding down, and our attention shifts to savoring the time that is left: we focus more on depth of experience, a small set of goals, a highly selected group of loved ones, and positive experience. We feel this in our bodies—the immediacy, fullness, and vibrancy of experience.

In my own writing on aging, I have emphasized our felt sense of having "less time ahead, more behind."[12] All the "time behind" helps us gain perspective, integrity, and wisdom, while the recognition that there is limited time ahead urges us to make the most of the time that is left. We can feel all the "time behind" embracing us and fortifying us. We can feel it strengthening our spines, sensitizing our hearts. At the same time, our recognition that there is "less time ahead" leads to a sense of urgency, a bodily pull to wake up and get moving. The foreshortened future leads to a pruning of our activities to include, as is possible, only the most crucial and enjoyable. To do all this, we have to hurry up and slow down at the same time! We have more of a sense of "cutting to the chase." Why wait? What am I impelled to do in the time that remains?

In her delightful book *Growing Old*, French psychoanalyst Danielle Quinodoz also muses about how our sense of time changes as we get older.[13] Knowing that time is limited, she says, there can be a new and startling awareness of present time, "small seconds of eternity," in which we have access to another dimension of time that is nonlinear. As we get older, she says, we are able to dwell more often in "eternal time," as opposed to clock time. I think this is perhaps what my eighty-nine-year-old interviewee Mary was alluding to when she said, with a sly smile, "There's less time but also *more* time, because I can *take* time."

Sometimes, when we *take* time, a second of eternity, it feels like bliss. There is a fresh immediacy of experiencing, as if a veil has been removed. The sensory input can be overwhelming. I felt it lying in my sleeping bag in the open air under a vast sky white with stars in Death Valley. I felt it more recently when I went with a friend to Point Reyes National Seashore to celebrate her sixtieth birthday. As we walked along the magnificent path to Abbotts Lagoon, we suddenly found ourselves in a candescent, psychedelic landscape. Goldenbush, blue lupine, and poppy glistened around us. Scarlet ice plants glowed in the dunes. The scent of sagebrush was intoxicating. At the little beach, we tore off our shoes, curling and uncurling our toes in the warm sand. So much beauty, so much joy, a caesura in time.

Integrity

In our last stage of life, Erikson believed, our psychic energy is focused on achieving "integrity," without which we are likely to feel more "despair." By integrity, he meant the "acceptance of one's one and only life . . . a recognition that an individual life is the accidental coincidence of but one life cycle with but one segment of history . . . an emotional integration . . . and a final consolidation [in which] death loses its sting."[14] He is describing our radical acceptance of the person we have become and the life we have led and the recognition of our own "transience," without fear of death. We feel buoyed, Erickson says, by a sense of some "larger order" across time, culture, and generations.

In a similar manner, Quinodoz suggested that the most important task for the older therapy patient (or, I think, for *any* of us) is the reconstruction of our own internal life history, thus giving meaning to the whole of our life by integrating the past into the present. Quinodoz writes, "It's difficult to give up our place peacefully without first having found it . . . to leave life peacefully without first feeling that we have actually lived."[15]

I find myself thinking back on my younger years, thus bringing my earlier incarnations into the present, where I can reflect on them and feel my continuity with them. It is solidifying to feel my self-continuity over my life span. Even though I am older and, in some ways, different, I am also the same. I am more fully myself. At this age, I can be more realistic about myself. I know more about my own limitations, as well as the limitations of even the best relationships. In my twenties, I vaguely imagined I should be able to become or achieve anything I wanted. In my thirties, I became more aware of the boundaries imposed by my emotional, intellectual, and physical inheritance and life experience. That awareness has only increased with the years, bringing with it, yes, certain disappointments and wistfulness but also, more importantly, a sense of being able to use myself more fully as I *am* rather than as who I should be. I know now that I do best when I go with the river rather than against it. There is less often a "they" that knows more than I do. I can wake up to who I am now, in both mind and body, who I want to be *now*.

I think this is what so many of my interviewees were saying when they described feeling "more like myself" as they got older. In fact, the older the interviewee was, the more she tended to feel more like herself. A very positive trend! People talked about giving up illusions and stories about themselves, throwing off the veils, coming out of hiding, letting their faces and bodies *show* without the need for excessive cover-up or adornment. They described feeling greater freedom from the rules. They could more easily let go of how they should be, how their body should be, how life should be. One said: "What I think these days is, 'Here I am, like it or not.'"

Reba, a musician and my friend of almost fifty years, told me about a new fire in her belly:

> I feel more and more myself . . . more just not willing to shy away from my sensibilities. I'm finding my voice. I've always felt self-conscious about my words, about expressing myself. But now I'm starting to write down what I think. It's my voice—it doesn't matter how good it is. I just keep shaping it. If other people don't give a shit about my voice, it doesn't matter. It's my voice. It's like when you're learning a new piece of music, you just keep getting all those little tangles out and you just keep trying different things and the music gets more and more itself and suddenly Beethoven is standing in your living room. That's what I'm doing now, all the time, just following my voice; I don't need to ever be done.

Finding one's voice takes audacity, of course, which reminds me of Anaïs Nin, who said, "Life shrinks or expands according to one's courage."[16]

An essential part of integrity, to my mind, is the ability to really dwell in and feel "at one" with our bodies. And you know by now that I believe our capacity for mind-body integration, or embodiment, increases as we age. The lessening of our sensory, hormonal, and emotional reactivity helps us sense ourselves more deeply and pleasurably—as I did to an extreme degree that blissful day at Point Reyes. But wait: Is this not a contradiction to feel our bodies *less* and *more* at the same time? No, I don't think so. Precisely because of our more muted bodily reactivity, including the absence of hormonal tumult, our bodies are slower and quieter. We can be calmer and more present in the moment, which allows us to more easily attend to the more refined sensations of our older bodies. Of course, all this becomes more difficult if we are in severe pain or enduring other serious disability.

Indeed, as we age, we learn to negotiate a dual relationship to our body, which involves both a letting go and a holding closer. As we ease up and finally let go of aspects of our "outside bodies" that may have been very important—like physical beauty, athletic prowess, or being an object of sexual desire—we free ourselves up to attach more profoundly to our "inside bodies." We develop a more tranquil, grounded sense of ourselves that comes with feeling our bodies from deep within.

Wisdom

I hesitated to include "wisdom" among the benefits of aging, because the concept is so overworn yet undefined, and because so many older people are certainly *not* wise. Yet I realize that there *is* something about older age that lends itself to being "wise" and that is worth thinking about. To me, wisdom grows out of experience, perspective, and maturity, but it is more than that. It involves vision, insight, perceptiveness—the ability to "see into" a particular situation or emotional conflict or the human condition so we get a sense of what's "really going on" and what might calm or enlighten all involved. Wisdom seems to grow out of the *integration* of our different faculties; we are more able to use body and brain, heart and mind, logical and holistic hemispheres of the brain at the same time.

We develop more of what I'll call *social wisdom*, which makes our interpersonal relationships easier in so many ways. Older people, studies show, use more complex reasoning that brings in multiple perspectives and compromise when faced with social dilemmas.[17] Being less quick to anger, we are better at dealing with charged emotional conflicts and at mediating interpersonal problems. We are more grateful, generous, understanding, tolerant. There is newfound sympathy, acceptance, and compassion for others. We are more invested in and satisfied with our relationships. We are kinder to our partners and tend to be kinder to each other. We are less likely to hold a grudge, more likely to forgive.[18]

We are more able to accept the realities of our lives. We can face difficult truths—like aging and death. In fact, I have a theory that lowering our defenses against mortality leads to a profound lowering of *all* our defenses.[19] If all fears are built around fear of death, as Ernest Becker said, and death anxiety is part of all anxiety, then, as we become more comfortable facing death, we also become more prepared to meet the other rudely unsettling challenges of life. Picture our defenses against facing our mortality as a much too large lid, one that covers not only death but all manner of feared, difficult, or overwhelming experiences. If we are able to take the lid off death, we may be more able to see and acknowledge our many other fears. Compared to fear of mortality, our other challenges can appear more like blips on the radar screen. We can more easily tolerate our mother's dementia or our friend's cancer or the narrowing of our spinal column or our son's impending divorce. If we are able to stay with our awareness of our own finitude, I believe we have lifted a major veil and can better accept "the way things are."

Psychoanalyst Elliott Jaques[20] pointed to a waning of "omnipotent" thinking ("I can do anything!") and greater humility in older age, which allows us to better tolerate dependency and to sustain love for the important people in our lives, despite their shortcomings. Calvin Colarusso, in his writings on life-span development, proposed a "fifth individuation" process in our last stages, in which we develop the ability to say good-bye to loved ones and to the world.[21] Indeed, our decreased emotional negativity and heightened acceptance and self-compassion may make it easier to say our good-byes. We have also been slowly building our "loss muscles" through multiple little good-byes over a lifetime.

Gisela Labouvie-Vief, an influential life-span psychologist at the University of Geneva in Switzerland, posits that as we age, we become more able to think with our hearts and minds simultaneously. Because we can more often use emotion to inform our thinking, we get deeper insight into ourselves and others, and we make better, more humane decisions.[22] Observations from many aging experts converge on additional qualities of wisdom that can emerge as we grow older, including being more honest, resilient, spiritual, courageous, and focused on the riches of the inner world and on "what matters most."

With increasing wisdom, we have a deepening understanding that "life is hard" for everyone, although, unfortunately, much more so for some. This realization allows us to more easily resonate with the troubles and irritating quirks of others with a sense of shared humanity. I often think of psychoanalyst Harry Stack Sullivan's comment, "We are all much more simply human than otherwise."[23] The gradual accretion of experience and understanding over the life span can give us more compassion. We become more able to tolerate the losses of the aging process. We become "sadder but wiser." We can move from a focus on who we were to who we're *becoming*.

Creativity

The conventional wisdom until quite recently was that the brain continues to degenerate as we age, upending our capacity for new, creative thinking. Happily, this is not the case! Our brains not only remain "plastic" into old age but also are capable of *creative, new thought*, even serious artistic productivity. Marian Diamond, the pioneering brain researcher who proved "neuroplasticity" (see chapter 1), also discovered that the brain stays flexible into older age and keeps on sprouting new connections. The brain continues to respond positively to what Diamond calls "challenge" by, for example, increasing the size of neuronal cell bodies and nuclei and thickening the cerebral cortex.[24] Use it or lose it. Diamond was her own best evidence. She remained one of the most popular professors at UC Berkeley (well-known on campus for carrying around a preserved human brain in a hatbox), until she retired at age eighty-seven.

Gene Cohen, geriatric psychiatrist and director of the Institute on Health, Humanities, and Aging at George Washington University, probably did more than anyone else to highlight and celebrate the unique creative power generated by age and experience. Cohen wrote: "Creativity can blossom at any age—and in fact, it can bloom with more depth and richness in older adults because it is informed by their vast stores of knowledge and experience."[25] Cohen's research also proved that creative activity is particularly good for the aging brain, because it furthers the brain's ability to grow, change, and form new connections.[26]

Examples of famous older creative people abound: Carl Jung completed his masterpiece and autobiography, *Memories, Dreams, Reflections*, at the age of eighty-five, the same year he died. Martha Graham danced until she was seventy-five and choreographed her last work at age ninety-six. Michelangelo was designing the dome of St. Peter's Basilica in Rome when he died at age eighty-eight.

And we don't have to be geniuses to be creative. The potential for creativity is alive in all of us as we age, if we make space for it. "Just as aging is a journey and not an end," Cohen wrote, "creativity is a process or an outlook, not a product. It is a distinctly human quality that exists independent of age and time, reflecting a deeper dimension of energy capable of transforming our lives at any age."[27]

This "deeper dimension of energy" is, I believe, to be found in the body. Creativity is animated by emotion, and, as you now know, emotion is grounded and experienced in the body. The colors and shapes of visual art, or the sounds and rhythm of music, translate our emotional experience into something we can see or hear with our senses. Creative activities also stimulate states of well-being, "flow," enhanced memory, better health, and even the production of protective immune cells.

I know I am in the presence of great art when my body responds before my mind. When I'm in a museum and come upon certain works by, for example, Mark Rothko, Gerhard Richter, or Claude Monet, I find myself stopping, falling into the paintings, gazing at them for a long time, then later coming back to gaze some more. It's definitely a body experience I'm after. I still remember being seized by Van Gogh's "Lilac Bush" thirty-five years ago at the Hermitage Museum in St. Petersburg and circling back to it again and again to re-experience the bodily delight of entering that glorious painting. When I think of Richard Wagner's opera *Tristan und Isolde*, I return to the body experience of something dark and exciting washing over me, like huge waves in the sea.

As I get older, I'm finding that my experience of art—whether music, painting, sculpture, or dance—is becoming ever more intense, because my body is quieter, slower, more open, more responsive. I'm not in a hurry. There is more time to let great beauty enter me, whether human-created or in nature. The intensity of experience is increasing. I can't imagine what it will be like if I live twenty more years.

A Gift of Dementia

There is an odd but wonderful coda to these thoughts on aging and creativity. It turns out that an uncommon form of dementia, which significantly impairs the frontotemporal lobe of the brain, can actually give rise to new or enhanced artistic skills! Bruce Miller, clinical director of the Memory and Aging Center at UCSF, studied a series of patients with dementia who started to express new musical or visual abilities as their dementia progressed.[28] One sixty-eight-year-old man began to compose classical music. Miller theorized that this man's musical abilities had been suppressed by the more dominant, cognitive part of his brain, and then, when the dominant part deteriorated, the musical part was released to express itself. How adaptable we humans are! If we lose our verbal pathways, we can access other channels of communication, other ways of creatively expressing who we are.

Morituri Salutamus

... For age is opportunity no less
Than youth itself, though in another dress,
And as the evening twilight fades away
The sky is filled with stars, invisible by day.

HENRY WADSWORTH LONGFELLOW

What Determines How Well We Age?

The benefits of aging I've been exploring describe positive *trends* among older people, but not what it's like for each individual. Each of us ages differently. Some will be happier or more aware than others, and some of us will be miserable. So, what helps to determine how good we feel during our later years? There are so many individual factors that affect us—temperament, upbringing, ability, emotional and physical health, socioeconomic level, life experience, luck, and so on—but most aging experts do agree on a few things that really do seem to help *all* of us age more comfortably.

There are three factors that the research demonstrates are vitally important for aging well: maintaining social connections, finding meaning and purpose, and cultivating healthy emotions, like gratitude. Exercise/movement, diet, and sleep are also crucially important, but since I covered them in the previous chapter I won't mention them again here.

Maintaining Social Connections

The famous Grant Study[29] of the Harvard Medical School has tracked 268 male Harvard students (including JFK) and 456 controls from Boston for seventy-five years. Around fifty-nine of them, mostly now in their nineties, are still in the study. The clearest message we get from this definitive study is that good relationships keep us happier and healthier throughout our lives and that loneliness can kill us.

Social connection is, in fact, a *necessary* condition for lasting happiness, according to a major positive psychology study.[30] The quality of your relationships at age fifty has a bigger effect than smoking or cholesterol level for health and memory at age eighty.[31] People who are more socially connected to family, friends, and communities live longer and are 60 percent less likely to develop dementia.[32] It turns out that interacting with others is among the most complex things we can do with our brains, so it keeps our brains and bodies in fine fettle.

Maintaining social connections is particularly important if you are one of the significant number of older people who struggle with loneliness, a serious condition that can harm your body as well as your psyche and decrease your life span.[33] The "Happiness Report," a joint project of the United Nations and Gallup that ranks different countries on happiness, consistently finds that the happiest countries are those that prioritize social connection and helping others, like Italy or India.

Finding Meaning and Purpose

Most of us are also happier, research shows, if we're working on something meaningful, whether it's paid work or artistic endeavors or volunteer projects that inspire us. What's important is to engage with a project that allows you to focus on your own particular deeply held *values*.

We human beings are happiest when we have a purpose. Novelist Barbara Kingsolver wrote, in *Animal Dreams*, "I've about decided that's the main thing that separates happy people from the other people. The feeling that you're a practical item, like a sweater or a socket wrench."[34] Between 25 and 40 percent of people who retire reenter the work force; when asked why, they cite needing a "sense of purpose," "using your brain," and "social engagement."[35] The best time to retire? Probably never. But you don't have to be doing paid work: you can be doing anything that rouses you out of bed in the morning.

There's also a new wrinkle (as it were). Our greatly increasing longevity has created new meaning-making challenges. We've added thirty years to our life expectancy over the past century, and those years have all been tacked on to our retirement phase, making it incredibly long and empty. We work like crazy during the middle stage so that we can finally ("whew!") retire and do what we want. But what *is* that? There really are no standard or prescribed "tasks" for our last phase (except for grandparenting, if we are lucky) as there have been for earlier phases. Valory Mitchell, coauthor of a recent study of life-span development, suggests how "lost" older people can feel: "It may appear that the river of life has flowed steadily along a clear channel, only to become lost in a marsh, where there is no clear direction, no visible current or riverbanks to contain it."[36]

We are fortunate, therefore, to have the unstoppable Laura Carstensen to creatively reenvision our life course in this age of increased longevity. If she had her way, she would spread things out and allow more years for education, apprenticeship, and starting families before full-time work begins at age forty, then diffuse work over the adult years, making work less hurried and stressful. We would still be midcareer in our fifties or sixties, slowly easing out of work during the last stage of life until we retire at eighty. However, we would *never* be expected to stop contributing.[37]

Not everyone wants to work until age eighty, however, and I don't want to disparage anyone who decides to spend her later years on the beach or the hiking trails or reading novels. I particularly don't want to blame unhappy older people for not aging "correctly." We find our meaning, purpose, and happiness in so many different ways.

Cultivating Healthy Emotions

While many of the pleasures of growing older unfold naturally as a result of lessened brain-body reactivity and more life experience, you can enjoy your older age even more if you *intentionally* work with your emotions, body, and behavior. Our miraculous capacity for neuroplasticity allows us to continually reshape our brains though new experiences. And, as you now know, it's possible to "cultivate" positive emotions through meditation and other practices that actually rewire your brain in ways that promote greater well-being.

In fact, positive psychologist Martin Seligman and others have shown conclusively that simply changing certain little, everyday *behaviors* can bring about dramatic changes in your well-being. Contrary to the American Dream, genuine happiness does not come mainly from your circumstances (perfect family, perfect job, good looks, lots of money) but from *what you do* and *who you are*.

Laurie Santos, a Yale psychology professor, whose course on happiness is one of the most popular in the university's history (and draws millions online, starting during the pandemic), offers various research-based "mental hacks"—behavioral shortcuts to changing your inner state.[38] For example, since research shows that social connection is a *necessary* condition for happiness in older age, you would be well-advised to bump up your social interactions. You can increase your sense of social connectedness in surprisingly simple ways, like texting a friend or talking with someone on the street or at the grocery store or the dog park. Santos calls happiness "a leaky tire" that you have to keep pumped up.

Gratitude and helping others, research shows, dramatically increase our well-being in older age and are particularly important to cultivate. One popular way to boost your sense of gratitude is to keep a "gratitude log" in which you write down three things you're grateful for every night. Another idea comes from a striking study by Seligman's group.[39] Participants were asked to write a letter to someone they were really grateful to have in their lives—but had not yet told. They were then asked to visit that person and read them the letter. What the researchers found was that the bump in happiness for the letter *writer* from this brief exercise could last as long as a month!

We also feel better when we lend a hand to others. When a friend calls after getting a scary medical diagnosis, you may not simply want to express your sympathy over the phone but, instead, might drop whatever you're doing and show up at her door with flowers. Research shows that helping others, even in the smallest of ways, benefits the helper even more than the helpee. One famous study found that money spent on others makes you happier than money spent on yourself.[40] Other positive emotions are also being widely studied and can be cultivated, as I discussed in chapter 4, including compassion, kindness, love, and awe.

Boosting Your Body Sense

Another way to age well, of course, is to increase your interoceptive awareness. I have chosen to focus on this so intensely because it has not been fully appreciated by other writers on aging. Building interoceptive aware-ness has not been given its due, in spite of research demonstrating its value and despite its being intuitively obvious that it is *exactly what an aging body needs*. As your physical body become less robust, stable, and reliable, the best corrective is to feel firmly rooted in your body, with those roots extending deep into the earth. As you become less "grounded" externally, you urgently need to feel more grounded *internally*. As you know, you can intentionally work on your sense of well-being directly *through* your body. When you deeply sense your body, you immediately know how to protect, care for, and enjoy it. It is one of the best ways I know to love yourself.

The Embodiment of Ageism

There is something else—pervasive, crafty, and insidious—that we have to come to terms with, in order to age well. We must learn to uncover and combat the negative age stereotypes still rife in our society. Ageism is a huge, underacknowledged contributor to our aging woes. Despite our current, vibrant national conversation about inclusion and equity for all races, ethnicities, genders, and sexual orientations, we have yet to effec-tively address *age inequality*.

Ageism, not just age, lives and breathes in our *bodies*. Our society's ageist messages get absorbed as our own ageist self-perceptions and body maladies. Our ageist beliefs about ourselves, even more than the aging pro-cess itself, can weaken our muscles, tighten our joints, stoop our shoulders, wobble our balance, dim our vision, muffle our ears, dull our attrac-tiveness, scramble our brains, and sap our energy. We internalize our culture's fear of and distaste for what's in store for all of us (if we're lucky), and ageism becomes literally embodied.

Ageism is also transmitted body to body. Like our minds, our bodies take their cues from the bodies we grow up with, which themselves express the habits of bodies in the surrounding culture. Our parent—particularly our mother if we are female—continually transmits her own feelings about her body to us, and we absorb her feelings as our own. Is our mother accept-ing of her older body, or does she hate it or feel alienated from it? My interviewee Kelly, age seventy-four, slowly shook her head as she said:

My mother suffered so with aging and had facelifts because of my Dad, who wanted someone younger. It was so hard to watch her in despair about getting older. She didn't talk about it, but I just knew, I could feel what she was going through, how hungry she was for compliments. And I felt guilty when she talked about me with all her friends about how beautiful I was . . . something I had that she had lost.

Because ageist beliefs reside partly in our bodies, they eclipse conscious thought, including our best intentions, principles, philosophies, desires, and needs. Remember, we must "*learn* to be old. . . . It is something we are initiated into . . . partly in response to the ways we are treated."[41] The internalization of aging stereotypes begins all the way back in our childhoods, when we adopt the attitudes and stereotypes of our family and cultural environment. Young children are already ageist: in one study, 66 percent of four- to seven-year-old children said they did not want to become old.[42] Unlike race and gender stereotypes, which we discover at the same time that we are developing group identities, we acquire age stereotypes decades before becoming old and, as a result, are more likely to automatically accept them without questioning their validity. Unfortunately, it is also true of age stereotypes that older people's views of older people are as negative as those of younger people.

Yale epidemiological researcher Becca Levy and her colleagues rocked the world of aging research two decades ago when they first provided startling scientific proof of the impact of negative aging stereotypes on *longevity*. She and her team found that older people who had more positive views of aging, which had been measured decades earlier, lived *seven-and-a-half years longer* than those with more negative views![43] More recently, another study by Levy's team found that older people who rejected age stereotypes were also much less likely to develop Alzheimer's.[44]

For both studies, Levy and her coauthors tracked the "self-perceptions of aging," measured twenty-three years earlier, of 660 individuals aged fifty or older, who were part of a large community-based survey (the Ohio Longitudinal Study of Aging and Retirement). They had been asked whether they agreed with popular stereotypes about aging, such as (in abbreviated form): (1) you lose your pep, (2) things get worse, (3) you are less useful, and (4) you are less happy. The researchers then compared the participants' scores on age stereotyping with recent survival data from the National Death Index and found that those with more positive views of aging increased their longevity by over seven years. How did Levy explain this? People with more negative views, she said, were more likely to view health care and exercise as futile so didn't do these self-care functions and, consequently, died earlier. The study also confirmed that aging stereotypes acquired earlier in life persist over time.

It gets even better. The participants' perceptions of aging, the researchers found, had a greater impact on longevity than gender, socioeconomic status, loneliness, or functional health! And when the results were compared to those of other studies of longevity, Levy's team found that positive self-perceptions of aging increased longevity more than low blood pressure, low cholesterol, BMI, nonsmoking, or exercise. Those with more positive age stereotypes (developed earlier in life) had a stronger "will to live" and were much less likely to experience a cardiovascular event over the next thirty-eight years. In another influential study of 598 men and women aged seventy years or older and interviewed over ten years, Levy and team found that older persons with positive age stereotypes were 44 percent more likely to fully recover from severe disability (measured by improvements in bathing, dressing, transferring, and walking).[45]

Clearly, the aging process can no longer be explained only as a physiological process of inevitable decline. Ageism is real, and it affects the body as well as the mind. In a 2001 survey of eighty-four people aged sixty or older by ageism scholar Erdman Palmore, nearly 80 percent reported experiencing ageism: for example, other people's assuming that they had age-related memory or physical impairments when they didn't.[46] The most frequent type of ageism, reported by 58 percent of respondents, involved being told jokes that poke fun at older people. Which doesn't mean they're not funny. "I know I'm getting old," said Joan Rivers. "I went to buy sexy underwear, and they automatically giftwrapped it."

Call to Action (not Bingo)

One thing that made Levy's studies of age stereotyping and longevity so persuasive is that they looked at clear, real-world outcomes. "If a virus was found to diminish life expectancy by over 7 years," writes Levy, "our society would certainly make every effort to identify the cause and treatment." You bet we would. So, what "treatment" does she prescribe for negative age stereotyping? "Our society needs to make a conscientious effort to delegitimize denigrating views of older people,"[47] she says, adding we must use the same strict standards of egalitarianism that are currently being applied to racism and sexism. Combatting ageism begins by looking inside ourselves and acknowledging our own internalized ageist views.

What if we became part of a movement to transform our society's vision of aging? Our generations have successfully advocated for the rights of women and for people of every color, sexual and gender orientation, and disability. But the movement for the dignity of the *aging*, the group to which we *all* may belong, is still in the Dark Ages. Isn't it time to put *age equality* on our nation's human rights agenda? Wouldn't it be wonderful if we could help create a different vision of aging, more like that in Asia, where older people are treated with tremendous respect and even celebration?

I think of a huge ceremony I attended at a temple in the Tamil Nadu region of southern India a few years ago. Hundreds of people, mainly family members of all ages, attended the event, feasting and dancing together as musicians drummed and played horns for hours on end. What were they celebrating? The Shashtiabda Poorthi, the "completion of the sixtieth year" (sixty-first birthday) of the patriarch of the family, as well as the renewal of the couple's marriage. This is a memorable turning point, a joyful introduction to the more spiritual, less worldly years to come. The beaming older couple stood with arms around each other in front of the huge crowd, as family member after family member knelt adoringly before them, placing garlands of white flowers around their necks and pouring holy water over them. This celebration of older age is the most important Hindu family celebration in this part of India.

To bring this kind of veneration and joyful celebration of older age to our Western countries, we need to start with ourselves. We ourselves must be *proud* of our age, as Gray Panther leader Maggie Kuhn used to say years ago. We need to present to the world a strong, proud, and embodied sense of ourselves. We need to say, in essence, here I am, an older person with deep understanding of how people and the world operate, with so much to offer and nothing to hide!

One of the primary complaints of the original *Our Bodies, Ourselves* activists in the early 1970s (remember them?) was how the medical profession treated symptoms without considering the *social context* of the illness.[48] The social context of many "symptoms" of aging is our dismal view of older people, and this is unfortunately true of the ways many doctors and other caregivers relate to older people. My seventy-seven-year-old friend Frannie, who recently sprained her knee hiking in the mountains at nine thousand feet elevation, complained to her doctor that her knee was not improving, and he *actually* said, "What do you expect at your age?" to which Frannie responded, "Well, my right one is just fine, thanks." Older people are still often called "honey" or talked to in baby talk or in overenunciated speech. And when I recently asked a young male clerk in the grocery store where the lentils were, he led me all the way across the store to point them out to me, when a simple "Aisle 3 on the right" would have sufficed. Similarly, too many adult children of older people make too many medical and legal decisions for Mom or Dad without seriously discussing it with them, as Atul Gawande sensitively describes in his book *Being Mortal*.

Like the first *Our Bodies, Ourselves* movement in the 1970s, our goals would be to champion realistic body acceptance and appreciation (including excellent self-care) and to lessen self-hatred and disgust. A pro-age movement must begin with getting to know, accept, and even cherish our actual flesh-and-blood bodies, messy and imperfect as they are. Such a movement could build upon the excellent work of the current body positivity movement in changing women's relationships to the beauty, fashion, and entertainment industries, as well as existing efforts to change women's participation in business, politics, childrearing, and other endeavors. There is also still plenty of room for change in women's relationships to men, especially those in power. As we become stronger, more embodied, and more self-aware, we effortlessly become part of a groundswell to change our society's vision of aging.

Reenvisioning Ourselves in Older Age

So, what can we actually *do* as individuals to move ourselves and our society forward? What comes to your mind? Here are a few of my favorite approaches:

- **Ferret out and combat negative age stereotyping.** Learn everything you can about how ageism manifests in our society. Make an effort to notice and acknowledge your own ageist beliefs and actions. Know that every one of us of every age is ageist to some degree, so you're in good company. Monitor the ways you are sending ageist messages to yourself and others. Are you lying about your age? Are you imagining people on the street feeling sorry for you because of your age? Are you imagining that younger people don't want to talk with you because you're boring to them? Try to speak to yourself differently.

  Keep on the lookout for ageist remarks. "You look really good for sixty-six." "Are you *still* working?" Observe romanticized, as well as derogatory, ageist stereotypes. Ever notice how older people in TV commercials are always smiling, smiling, smiling, as they ballroom dance in the kitchen? Who *does* that?

  What you hear from others and what you tell yourself *does* change how you feel about getting older, which can change your experience of aging—even the length of your life. If we shed our own ageism, we can break the cycle and spread our healthy acceptance of aging to our children and future generations.

- **Dump the image of the aging process as an "arc,"** which pictures us sliding down from the apex to our bleak later years. Imagine instead an endless, upward spiral with multiple trajectories.[49] See aging as culmination and fulfillment, rather than as epilogue or decline. Don't equate aging with disability, decay, or deterioration. Brains are continuously changing based on our experience—that is, changed by life itself. We can change our brains and our bodies. We can change our lives.

Some people, like me, want to go on working "forever" in their chosen field. Some can't wait to retire from their "day job" and devote themselves to a serious new artistic pursuit. Others get the most pleasure from taking care of their grandchildren. Some want to spend their days hiking and biking. Some want to dedicate themselves to social action to better society. Others want to spend days playing bridge or in the pool. There is no right way. When you imagine that upward spiral, what different trajectories do you see for yourself?

- **Join "age awareness" groups or classes.** Join or create your own consciousness-raising groups, only this time focused on *age*-consciousness. My old friend Linda Blachman, a facilitator of mindfulness-based Wise Aging groups, says, "I try to help women navigate all the ongoing *transitions* of aging, like changes in health and appearance, caregiving and relationship loss, retirement and legacy, work and creativity, meaning and spirituality. . . . It really helps to go through all this with other people!"

- **Engage in intergenerational activities.** Engage with people significantly older and younger than you are by purposely making intergenerational friendships and pursuing intergenerational activities. Gyms and libraries are places where this already happens to some extent. The AARP Foundation has a program called Experience Corps that matches older adult tutors with economically disadvantaged children. It turns out that the program not only helps the kids but also helps the older volunteers, even increasing their brain function in the hippocampus and cortex.[50] Try to educate your workplace or other companies about the importance of retaining and integrating older employees. Multigenerational teams, research shows, outperform single-generational ones.

- **Pursue body awareness classes or activities.** I have not been reticent about encouraging you to develop your body awareness! You are by now familiar with the reams of research showing how body practices can dramatically change your emotional and physical well-being in older age. As you move through these last phases of your life, you have another opportunity to reconnect mind and body and create a healthier relationship with your body. It's never too late to begin.

- **Offer your own gifts to the world.** When society acts as if we have nothing to offer, we have to stand up and offer our own energy and skills to the world. We teach an art class. We open a tiny café. We help kids learn to write. We do accounting for our church or temple. Our greater positivity and emotional steadiness make us excellent candidates to serve as facilitators of various groups. We older people have to make sure that we get the respect and the audience we deserve.

We should also offer opportunities for meaningful work or activities to *other* older people. Let's train ourselves to sometimes think first of older people when there's a job to be done. Sidelining older people comes with a huge cost in lost economic and creative productivity and the unique wisdom and experience that comes from a long life.

When Gloria Steinem was eighty-four she was asked, "Who are you passing the torch to?" She answered, laughing, "I'm not giving up my torch, thank you! I'm using my torch to light other people's torches. . . . If we each have a torch, there's a lot more light."[51] Absolutely. As we get older, we don't want to hand off our torch to others; we want to continue to light our own way ahead. Who knows what we have yet to illuminate?

I leave you with some reminders for how to forge a healthier relationship with your older body:

- Allow yourself to feel awestruck by the miracle of your body in all its complexity and magnificence.

- Understand that your mind, your emotions, and your very sense of self are deeply rooted in your body, so the future of "you" depends on listening to and taking care of your body.

- Remember that your body was "made" in and through relationship and continues to be remade and revised through relationship, so stay connected to others in an embodied way as much as you can.

- Know that you can keep on learning to sense and feel your body more through practice and training.

- Understand the scientific benefits of increasing your body awareness, including better emotional regulation, greater empathy for others, firmer emotional "boundaries," and more overall happiness.

- Recognize that ageism alters and damages our bodies as well as our minds, so work to root out and delegitimize ageist beliefs.

- Appreciate that by becoming more embodied, you can keep on *revising* your sense of your body and yourself until the very end.

- Deeply comprehend that you are part of nature, which, like you, is always aging.

This I know: when we live deeply grounded in our body, sensing ourselves from within, while maintaining a realistically positive view of our older years, we will age with more comfort, vibrancy, and joy. In fact, if we lovingly inhabit, care for, and enjoy our aging body, we can feel *better* in many ways in older age than we did when we were younger. We can finally make friends with our body, just as it is. So, sink down deep inside yourself, sense the rising and falling of your breath, and enjoy the humming aliveness of your body as a whole. Feel the loosening, the warmth, the strength, the *knowing* of being in your body—because it is *who you really are*.

Notes

Introduction

1. US Census Bureau, "Quick Facts," June 25, 2020, census.gov.

2. Valory Mitchell, "Who Am I Now?," *Women and Therapy* 32 (2009): 298–312, doi.org/10.1080/02703140902851930.

3. Wislawa Szymborska, quoted in Edward Hirsch, "A Poetry That Matters," *New York Times Magazine*, December 1, 1996, nytimes.com.

4. A. D. (Bud) Craig, *How Do You Feel?* (Princeton, NJ: Princeton University Press, 2016); Antonio Damasio, *The Feeling of What Happens* (New York: Houghton Mifflin Harcourt, 1999); Noga Arikha, "The Interoceptive Turn," *Aeon*, June 6, 2019, aeon.co.

5. Susie Orbach, *Bodies* (London: Picador, 2009).

6. American Society of Plastic Surgeons, "New Statistics Reflect the Changing Face of Plastic Surgery," plasticsurgery.org/news/press-releases/new-statistics-reflect-the-changing-face-of-plastic-surgery.

7. Ram Dass, *Still Here* (New York: Riverhead Books, 2000), 14.

8. Nicholas Bakalar, "Happiness May Come with Age, Study Says," *New York Times,* May 31, 2010, nytimes.com; Laura Carstensen, *A Long Bright Future* (New York: Public Affairs, 2009).

9. Susan Sands, "Less Time Ahead, More Behind," *Women and Therapy* 32 (2009): 158–69, doi.org/10.1080/02703140902851948.

Chapter 1. Living in the Body

1. Cristin Runfola, Ann Von Holle, Christine Peat et al., "Characteristics of Women with Body Size Dissatisfaction at Midlife," *Journal of Women and Aging* 4 (2013): 287–304, doi.org/10.1080 /08952841.2013.816215.

2. Patrick Kiger, "Older Americans Are Having More Cosmetic Surgery," AARP, June 15, 2018, aarp.org.older-plastic-surgery-botox-facelifts.

3. Jonathan Rauch, *The Happiness Curve* (New York: Picador, 2019).

4. Adrienne Harris, "Psychic Envelopes and Sonorous Baths," in *Relational Perspectives on the Body*, ed. Lewis Aron and Frances Anderson (New York: Routledge, 1998).

5. Susan Sands, "Body Experience in the Analysis of the Older Woman," *Psychoanalytic Inquiry* 40, no. 3 (2020): 173–88, doi.org /10.1080/07351690.2020.1727208; Susan Sands, "Eating Disorders Treatment as a Process of Mind-Body Integration," *Clinical Social Work Journal* 44, no. 1 (2016): 27–37, doi.org/10.1007/ s10615-015-0540-7.

6. Alan Fogel, *Body Sense* (New York: W. W. Norton, 2009).

7. Robert Stolorow and George Atwood, *Contexts of Being* (Hillsdale, NJ: Analytic Press, 1992).

8. Peter Oberg, "The Absent Body," *Aging and Society* 16, no. 6 (1996): 701–19, doi.org/10.1017/S0144686X00020055.

9. Sigmund Freud, "The Ego and the Id" (1923), in *The Standard Edition of the Complete Psychological Works of Sigmund Freud*, ed. J. Strachey (London: Hogarth, 1961), 19, 3–68.

10. Lewis Aron and Frances Anderson, eds., *Relational Perspectives on the Body* (New York: Routledge, 1998).

11. David Garner, Paul Garfinkel, Donald Schwartz, et al., "Cultural Expectations of Thinness in Women," *Psychological Reports* 47, no. 2 (1980): 483–91, doi.org/10.2466/pr0.1980.47.2.483.

12. Sandra Blakeslee and Matthew Blakeslee, *The Body Has a Mind of Its Own* (New York: Random House, 2008).

13. Charles Scott Sherrington coined the term "interoception" in the early twentieth century, but he was mainly referring to sensations from the viscera only. Some research on interoception appeared in the 1980s and 1990s, but the subject didn't really explode until the twenty-first century.

14. A. D. (Bud) Craig, *How Do You Feel?* (Princeton, NJ: Princeton University Press, 2016).

15. Antonio Damasio, *The Feeling of What Happens* (New York: Houghton Mifflin Harcourt, 1999).

16. Daniel Kahneman, *Thinking, Fast and Slow* (New York: Farrar, Straus & Giroux, 2011); Mark Sohms and Oliver Turnbull, *The Brain and the Inner World* (New York: Other Press, 2002).

17. John-Dylan Haynes, "Unconscious Decisions in the Brain," Max Planck Geselschaft, 2008, mpg.de/research/unconscious-decisions -in-the-brain.

18. Francisco Varela, Evan Thompson, and Eleanor Rosch, *The Embodied Mind* (Cambridge, MA: MIT Press, 1991).

19. Peter Fonagy and Mary Target, "The Rooting of the Mind in the Body," *Journal of the American Psychoanalytic Association* 55, no. 2 (2007): 411–56, doi.org/10.1177/00030651070550020501.

20. Qiyang Gao, Xianjie Ping, and Wei Chen, "Body Influences on Social Cognition Through Interoception," *Frontiers in Psychology* 10 (September 2019), doi.org/10.3389/fpsyg.2019.02066.

21. Blakeslee and Blakeslee, *The Body Has a Mind of Its Own.*

22. Marian Diamond, David Krech, and Mark Rosenzweig, "The Effects of an Enriched Environment on the Histology of the Rat Cerebral Cortex," *Journal of Comparative Neurology* 123, no. 4 (1964), doi.org/10.1002/cne.901230110.

23. Eleanor Maguire et al., "London Taxi Drivers and Bus Drivers," *Hippocampus* 16, no. 12 (2006): 1091–1101, doi.org/10.1002/hipo.20233.

24. Janina Boyke, "Training-Induced Brain Changes in the Elderly," *Journal of Neuroscience* 28, no. 28 (July 9, 2008): 7031–35, doi.org/10.1523/JNEUROSCI.0742-08.2008.

25. Elizabeth Blackburn, "Stress, Telomeres, and Telomerase in Humans," ibiology.org, YouTube, July 6, 2012.

26. Elizabeth Blackburn and Elissa Epel, *The Telomere Effect* (New York: Grand Central Publishing, 2018).

27. Sara Lazar et al., "Meditation Experience Is Associated with Increased Cortical Thickness," *Neuroreport* 16, no. 17 (2005), ncbi.nim.nih.gov.

Chapter 2. Triumphing Over the Body

1. Margaret Cruikshank, *Learning to Be Old: Gender, Culture, and Aging* (Lanham, MD: Rowman & Littlefield, 2009), 2.

2. Mike Featherstone and Mike Hepworth, "The Mask of Aging and the Post-Modern Life Course," in *The Body: Social Process and Cultural Theory*, ed. M. Featherstone, M. Hepworth, and B. Turner (London: Sage, 1991).

3. Todd Nelson, "Ageism: Prejudice Against Our Feared Future Self," *Journal of Social Issues* 61 (2005): 207–22, doi.org/10.1111/j.1540-4560.2005.00402.x.

4. Ashton Applewhite, *This Chair Rocks: A Manifesto Against Ageism* (New York: Celadon, 2016), 19.

5. Nora Ephron, *I Feel Bad About My Neck, and Other Thoughts on Being a Woman* (New York: Knopf, 2007), 5

6. Simone de Beauvoir, *The Second Sex* (New York: Knopf, 1949).

7. Simone de Beauvoir, *The Coming of Age* (New York: W. W. Norton, 1970).

8. Susan Sontag, "The Double Standard of Aging," *The Other Within Us* (New York: Routledge, 1972).

9. Sigrid Nunez, *What Are You Going Through?* (New York: Penguin, 2020), 52.

10. Susan Jacoby, *Never Say Die: The Myth and Marketing of the New Old Age* (New York: Vintage, 2012).

11. Jacoby, *Never Say Die*, 62.

12. Christopher Lasch, *The Culture of Narcissism: American Life in an Age of Diminishing Expectations* (New York: W. W. Norton, 1991).

13. Nicholas St. Fleur, Chloe Williams, and Charlie Wood, "Can We Live to 200?" *New York Times Magazine*, April 30, 2021, nytimes.com.

14. Anti-ageism task force at the International Longevity Center, "Ageism in America," 25, 2005, mailman.columbia.edu/sites /default/files/Ageism_in_America.pdf.

15. US Government National Institutes of Health, "Quick Statistics Compiled by the National Institute on Deafness and Other Communication Disorders (NIDCD)," nidcd.nih.gov/health/statistics /Pages/quick.aspx.

16. Randy Lilleston, "Joint Replacement Patients Getting Younger," *AARP: Health Conditions and Treatments*, March 9, 2018, aarp.org.

17. Calvin Colarusso, "Separation-Individuation Phenomena in Adulthood: General Concepts and the Fifth Individuation," *Journal of the American Psychoanalytic Association* 48, no. 4 (2000): 306.

18. Ernest Becker, *The Denial of Death* (New York: Free Press, 1973), ix.

19. Sigmund Freud, "On Transience," in *The Standard Edition of the Complete Psychological Works of Sigmund Freud*, ed. J. Strachey (London: Hogarth, 1961), 303–07.

20. William James, *The Principles of Psychology*, vol. 1 (New York: Henry Holt, 1890).

21. Hedda Bolgar, film interview, *The Beauty of Aging*, Laurie Schur, director/producer, 2006, beautyofaging.com.

22. James Baldwin, "As Much Truth as One Can Bear," *New York Times Book Review*, January 14, 1962.

23. Mary Pipher, *Women Rowing North* (New York: Bloomsbury, 2015).

24. Anne Karpf, *How to Age* (New York: Picador, 2014).

25. May Sarton, *At Seventy: A Journal* (New York: W. W. Norton, 1984).

26. Karpf, *How to Age*.

27. Buddhaghosa, *The Path of Purification (Visuddhimagga)*, trans. Bhikkhu Nanamoli (Onalaska, WA: Pariyatti Publishing, 1999).

28. Carlo Castaneda, *The Teachings of Don Juan* (Berkeley: University of California Press, 1969).

29. Tara Brach, *Radical Compassion* (New York: Penguin Life, 2020).

30. Ram Dass, *Still Here* (New York: Riverhead Books, 2000).

31. Lewis Richmond, *Aging as a Spiritual Practice* (New York: Gotham, 2012).

Chapter 3. The "Making" of the Body

1. Aikaterini Fotopoulou and Manos Tsakiris, "Mentalizing Homeostasis: The Social Origins of Interoceptive Inference," *Neuropsychoanalysis* 19, no. 1 (2017): 3–28, doi.org/10.1080/15294145.2017.1294031.

2. Hakan Olausson et al., eds., *Affective Touch and the Neurophysiology of CT Afferents* (New York: Springer, 2016).

3. J. Botvinick and J. Cohen, "Rubber Hands 'Feel' Touch That Eyes See," *Nature* 391 (1998): 756, doi.org/10.1038/35784.

4. Fotopoulou and Tsakiris, "Mentalizing Homeostasis."

5. Sigmund Freud, "The Ego and the Id" (1923), in *The Standard Edition of the Complete Psychological Works of Sigmund Freud*, ed. J. Strachey (London: Hogarth, 1961).

6. Donald Winnicott, "Mind in Its Relation to the Psyche-Soma" (1949), in *Through Pediatrics to Psychoanalysis* (New York: Basic, 1975), 243–54.

7. Donald Winnicott, *Human Nature* (New York: Routledge, 1970).

8. Esther Bick, "The Experience of the Skin in Early Object Relations," *International Journal of Psycho-Analysis* 49 (1968): 484–86.

9. Didier Anzieu, *The Skin Ego* (London: Routledge, 1985).

10. Wilfred Bion, *Learning from Experience* (London: Karnac, 1962).

11. David Linden, *Touch: The Science of Hand, Heart, and Mind* (New York: Penguin, 2015).

12. Virginia Hughes, "'Kangaroo Mothers' and the Power of Touch," *National Geographic*, October 10, 2013, phenomena.nationalgeographic .com/ . . . /kangaroo-mothers-and-the-power-of-touch.

13. Cleveland Clinic, "Kangaroo Care," 2018, my.clevelandclinic.org /health/treatments/12578-kangaroo-care.

14. Bion, *Learning from Experience.*

15. Heinz Kohut, *The Restoration of the Self* (New York: International Universities Press, 1977).

16. Robert Stolorow, Bernard Brandshaft, and George Atwood, *Psychoanalytic Treatment: An Intersubjective Approach* (Hillsdale, NJ: Analytic Press, 1987).

17. Giacomo Rizzolatti, Leonardo Fogassi, and Vittorio Gallese, "Neurophysiological Mechanisms Underlying the Understanding and Imitation of Action," *Nature Reviews Neuroscience* 2 (2001): 661–70, doi.org/10.1038/35090060.

18. Vittorio Gallese, "Embodied Simulation: From Neurons to Phenomenological Experience," *Phenomenology and the Cognitive Sciences* 4 (2005): 23–48.

19. Marian Diamond, David Krech, and Mark Rosenzweig, "The Effects of an Enriched Environment on the Histology of the Rat Cerebral Cortex," *Journal of Comparative Neurology* 123, no. 4 (1964), doi.org/10.1002/cne.901230110.

20. Daniel Stern, *The Interpersonal World of the Infant* (New York: Basic, 1985).

21. Richard Held and Alan Hein, "Movement-Produced Stimulation in the Development of Visually-Guided Behavior," *Journal of Comparative Physiological Psychology* 57, no. 5 (1963), doi.org/10.1037/h0040546.

22. Blandine Bril and Colette Sabatier, "The Cultural Context of Motor Development: Postural Manipulations in the Daily Life of Bambara Babies (Mali)," *International Journal of Behavioral Development* 9, no. 4 (1986), doi.org/10.1177/016502548600900403.

23. Seth Pollak et al., "Neurodevelopmental Effects of Early Deprivation in Post-Institutionalized Children," *Child Development* 81, no. 1 (2010): 224–36, doi.org/10.1111/j.1467-8624.2009.01391.x.

24. Susie Orbach, *Bodies* (London: Picador, 2009).

25. Susie Orbach and members of the BODI Group, "The Acquisition of a Body," in *Body-States*, ed. Jean Petrucelli (New York: Routledge, 2015).

26. Elizabeth Halsted, "Stretched to the Limit,'" in *Body-States*, ed. Jean Petrucelli (New York: Routledge, 2015), 82.

27. Eric Stice and Heather Shaw, "Role of Body Dissatisfaction in the Onset and Maintenance of Eating Pathology," *Journal of Psychosomatic Research* 53, no. 5 (2002): 985–93, doi.org/10.1016/S0022-3999(02)00488-9.

28. Professional Association for Childcare and Early Years (PACEY), *News*, August 21, 2016, pacey.org.uk.

29. Barbara Strauch, *The Primal Teen* (New York: Anchor, 2003).

30. Barbara Parry, "Special Issues in Menopause and Major Depressive Disorder," *Psychiatric Times* 30, no. 9 (September 2013).

31. Sarah Manguso, "Where Are All the Books About Menopause?" *New Yorker*, June 24, 2019, newyorker.com.

Chapter 4. The Emotional Body

1. A. D. (Bud) Craig, *How Do You Feel?* (Princeton, NJ: Princeton University Press, 2016); Antonio Damasio, *The Feeling of What Happens* (New York: Houghton Mifflin Harcourt, 1999).

2. Damasio, *The Feeling of What Happens*; Antonio Damasio, *Self Comes to Mind* (New York: Vintage, 2010).

3. Emeran Mayer, *The Mind-Gut Connection* (New York: Harper Wave, 2016).

4. Antonio Damasio and Gil Carvalho, "The Nature of Feelings: Evolutionary and Neurobiological Origins," *Nature Reviews Neuroscience* 14 (February 2013): 150, nature/reviews/neuro.

5. Anil Seth, Keisuke Suzuki, and Hugo Critchley, "An Interoceptive Predictive Coding Model of Conscious Presence," *Frontiers Psychology* 2 (2011): 395, doi.org/10.3389/fpsyg.2011.00395; Lisa Barrett, *How Emotions Are Made* (Boston: Houghton Mifflin Harcourt, 2017).

6. Pixar/Disney, *Inside Out* (2010).

7. Jack Panksepp and Lucy Biven, *The Archaeology of Mind* (New York: W. W. Norton, 2012); Mark Solms and Oliver Turnbull, *The Brain and the Inner World* (New York: Other Press, 2002).

8. Lisa Barrett, "You Aren't at the Mercy of Your Emotions," TED talk, January 17, 2018, youtube.com.

9. Aikaterini Fotopoulou and Manos Tsakiris, "Mentalizing Homeostasis: The Social Origins of Interoceptive Inference," *Neuropsychoanalysis* 19, no. 1 (2017): 3–28, doi.org/10.1080/15294145.2017.1294031.

10. Noam Shpancer, "Laws of Emotional Mastery," *Psychology Today*, May 4, 2021, psychologytoday.com/us/articles/202105/laws-emotional-mastery.

11. Dacher Keltner and Jonathan Haidt, "Approaching Awe, a Moral, Spiritual, Aesthetic Emotion," *Cognition and Emotion* 17, no. 2 (2003): 297–314, doi.org/10.1080/02699930302297.

12. Hugo Critchley, Stefan Wiens, Pia Rotshtein, et al., "Neural Systems Supporting Interoceptive Awareness," *Nature Neuroscience* 7 (2004): 189–95, nature.com/natureneuroscience.

13. Wolf Mehling, Cynthia Price, Jennifer Daubenmier et al., "The Multidimensional Assessment of Interoceptive Awareness (MAIA)," *PLOS ONE* 7, no. 11 (2012), doi.org/10.1371/journal .pone.0048230.

14. Aida Grabauskaite, Mindaugas Baranauskas, and Inga Griskova-Bulanova, "Interoception and Gender: What Aspects Should We Pay Attention To?" *Conscious Cognition* 48 (February 2017): 129–37, doi.org/10.1016/j.concog.2016.11.002.

15. Louann Brizendine, *The Female Brain* (New York: Morgan Road Books, 2006).

16. Tanya Singer, Ben Seymour, John O'Doherty et al., "Empathy for Pain Involves the Affective but Not Sensory Components of Pain," *Science* 303, no. 5661 (February 20, 2004): 1167–72, doi.org/10 .1126/science.1093535.

17. Fotopoulou and Tsakiris, "Mentalizing Homeostasis."

18. Christian Keysers, *The Empathic Brain* (Amsterdam: Social Brain Press, 2011).

19. Sally Olderbak, Claudia Sassenrath, Johannes Keller et al., "An Emotion-Differentiated Perspective on Empathy with the Emotion Specific Empathy Questionnaire," *Frontiers in Psychology* (July 1, 2014), doi.org/10.3389/fpsyg.2014.00653.

20. Wilma Bucci, "Emotional Communication in the Case of Antonio," *Psychoanalytic Inquiry* 38, no. 7 (2018): 518–29, doi.org /10.1080/07351690.2018.1504581; Jon Sletvold, *The Embodied Analyst* (New York: Routledge, 2014).

21. Laura Carstensen, *A Long Bright Future* (New York: Public Affairs, 2009).

22. Leanne Williams et al., "The Mellow Years? Neural Basis of Improving Emotional Stability over Age," *Journal of Neuroscience* 26, no. 24 (June 2006): 6422–30, doi.org/10.1523/neurosci.0022-06.2006.

23. J. T. Cacioppo, G. G. Berntson, A. Bechara, et al., "Could an Aging Brain Contribute to Subjective Well-Being? The Value Added by a Social Neuroscience Perspective," in *Social Neuroscience: Toward Understanding the Underpinnings of the Social Mind*, ed. A. Todorov, S. T. Fiske, and D. A. Prentice (Oxford: Oxford University Press, 2011), 249–62.

24. Williams et al., "The Mellow Years?"; Angela Gutchess, *Cognitive and Social Neuroscience of Aging* (Cambridge: Cambridge University Press, 2019).

25. Sahib Khalsa, David Rudrauf, and Daniel Tranel, "Interoceptive Awareness Declines with Age," *Psychophysiology* 46, no. 6 (2009): 1130–46, doi:10.1111/j.1469-8986.2009.00859.x; Jennifer Murphy, Hayley Geary, Edward Millgate, et al., "Direct and Indirect Effects of Age on Interoceptive Accuracy and Awareness Across the Adult Lifespan," *Psychonomic Bulletin Review* 25, no. 3 (2018): 1193–1202, doi.org/10.3758/s13423-017-1339-z.

26. Mai Mikkelsen et al., "Emotional Reactivity and Interoceptive Sensitivity: Exploring the Role of Age," *Psychonomic Bulletin and Review* 26 (2019): 1440–48, doi.org/10.3758/s13423-019-01603-y; Wendy Berry Mendes, "Weakened Links Between Mind and Body in Older Age: The Case for Maturational Dualism in the Experience of Emotion," *Emotion Review* 2, no. 3 (2010): 240–44, doi.org/10.1177/1754073910364149.

27. Jennifer MacCormack et al., "Aging Bodies, Aging Emotions," *Emotion* 21, no. 2 (2021): 227–46, doi.org/10.1037/emo0000699.

28. Sahib Khalsa, interview with author, July 1, 2020.

Chapter 5. Moving from Outside to Inside

1. Boston Women's Health Collective, *Our Bodies, Ourselves* (New York: Simon and Schuster, 1973).

2. Susie Orbach, *Bodies* (London: Picador, 2009), 8.

3. Luxury Activist, "Top Models Body Mass Index—Health Red Alert!" January 8, 2017, luxuryactivist.com.

4. Centers for Disease Control/National Center for Health Statistics, "Mean Body Weight, Height, Waist Circumference, and Body Mass Index Among Adults: United States, 1999–2000 Through 2015–2016," December 20, 2018, cdc.gov.

5. Thomas Cash, "Body Image: Past, Present, and Future," *Body Image* 1, no. 1 (2004), doi.org/10.1016/S1740-1445(03)00011-1.

6. Cristin Runfola, Ann Von Holle, Sara Trace et al., "Body Dissatisfaction in Women Across the Lifespan: Results of the UNC-SELF and Gender and Body Image (GABI) Studies," *European Eating Disorders Review* 21, no. 1 (2013): 52–59, doi.org/10.1002/erv .2201.

7. Kathryn Jackson et al., "Body Image Satisfaction and Depression in Midlife Women: The Study of Women's Health Across the Nation (SWAN)," *Archives of Women's Mental Health* 17, no. 3 (2014): 177–87, doi.org/10.1007/s00737-014-0416-9.

8. David Garner, Paul Garfinkel, Donald Schwartz, et al., "Cultural Expectations of Thinness in Women," *Psychological Reports* 47, no. 2 (1980): 483–91, doi.org/10.2466/pr0.1980.47.2.483.

9. Frances Bozsik and Brooke Bennett, *The Conversation*, 2018, theconversation.com.

10. Amy Brausch and Jennifer Muelenkamp, "Body Image and Suicidal Ideation in Adolescents," *Body Image* 4, no. 2 (2007): 207–12, doi.org/10.1016/j.bodyim.2007.02.001.

11. Vanessa Caceres, "Eating Disorders Statistics," *US News and World Report*, February 14, 2020, usnews.com.

12. David Garner and Ann Kearney Cooke, "Body Image in America: Survey Results," *Psychology Today*, February 1997, psychologytoday.com.

13. Hannah Borowsky et al., "Feminist Identity, Body Image, and Disordered Eating," *Eating Disorders* 24, no. 4 (2016): 297–311, doi.org/10.1080/10640266.2015.1123986.

14. Sarah Murnen and Linda Smolak, "Are Feminist Women Protected from Body Image Problems?," *Sex Roles: A Journal of Research* 60, nos. 3–4 (2009): 186–97, doi.org/10.1007/S11199-0089523-2.

15. Hannah Quittkat et al., "Body Dissatisfaction, Importance of Appearance, and Body Appreciation in Men and Women over the Lifespan," *Frontiers in Psychiatry* 10, no. 864 (December 2019), doi.org/10.3389/fpst.2019.00864; Trisha Pruis and Jeri Janowsky, "Assessment of Body Image in Younger and Older Women," *Journal of General Psychology* 137, no. 3 (2010): 225–38, doi.org/10.1080/00221309.2010.4844446.

16. Marika Tiggemann, "Body Image Across the Adult Life Span," *Body Image* 1, no. 1 (2004): 29–41, doi.org/10.1016/S17401445(03)00002-0.

17. Marika Tiggemann and Alice McCourt, "Body Appreciation in Adult Women: Relationships with Age and Body Satisfaction," *Body Image* 10, no. 4 (2013): 624–27, doi.org/10.1016/jbodyim.07.003.

18. Laura Avalos, Tracy Tylka, and Nichole Wood-Barcalow, "The Body Appreciation Scale: Development and Psychometric Evaluation," *Body Image* 2 (2005): 285–97, doi.org/10.1016/JBODYIM.2005.06.002.

19. Lewis Aron, "The Clinical Body and the Reflexive Mind," in *Relational Perspectives on the Body*, ed. Lewis Aron and Francis Sommer Anderson (New York: Routledge, 2009).

20. Barbara Fredrickson and Tomi-Ann Roberts, "Objectification Theory," *Psychology of Women Quarterly* 21, no. 2 (1997): 173–206, doi.org/10.1111/j.1471-6402.1997.tb00108.x.

21. Sarah Miller, "The Diet Industrial Complex Got Me, and It Will Never Let Me Go," *New York Times*, Style section, February 26, 2020, nytimes.com.

22. Tracy Tylka and Nichole Wood-Barcalow, "What Is and What Is Not Positive Body Image?," *Body Image* 14 (2015): 118–29, doi .org/10.1016/j.bodyim.2015.04.001.

23. Susan Sands, "Eating Disorders and Female Development," in *Dimensions of Self Experience: Progress in Self Psychology*, vol. 5, ed. Arnold Goldberg (Hillsdale, NJ: Analytic Press, 1989): 75–103, psycnet.apa.org; Susan Sands, "Bulimia, Dissociation, and Empathy," in *Psychodynamic Treatment of Anorexia Nervosa and Bulimia*, ed. Craig Johnson (New York: Guilford, 1991), 34–50, psycnet.apa.org; Susan Sands, "The Subjugation of the Body in Eating Disorders," *Psychoanalytic Psychology* 20: 103–116, psycnet .apa.org; Susan Sands, "Eating Disorders Treatment as a Process of Mind-Body Integration," *Clinical Social Work Journal* 44, no. 1 (2016): 27–37, doi.org/10.1007s10615-015-0540-7.

24. K. Pike and J. Rodin, "Mothers, Daughters, and Disordered Eating," *Journal of Abnormal Psychology* 100, no. 2 (1991): 198–204, psycnet.apa.org.

25. Hilde Bruch, *Eating Disorders: Obesity, Anorexia Nervosa, and the Person Within* (New York: Basic, 1973).

26. Claudia Goldin, "A Grand Gender Convergence: Its Last Chapter," *American Economic Review* 104, no. 4 (April 2014): 1091–1119, doi.org10.1257/aer.104.4.1091.

27. D. Badoud and M. Tsakiris, "From the Body's Viscera to the Body's Image: Is There a Link Between Interoception and Body Image Concerns?" *Neuroscience Biobehavioral Review* 77 (June 2017): 237–46, doi.org/10.1016/j.neubiorev.2017.03.017; Beate Herbert and Olga Pollatos, "The Body in the Mind: On the Relationship Between Interoception and Embodiment," *Topics in Cognitive Science* 4, no. 4 (2012): 692–704, doi.org/10.111/j .1756-8765.2012.01189.x.

28. Angela Wagner et al., "Altered Insula Response to Taste Stimuli in Individuals Recovered from Restricting Type Anorexia Nervosa," *Neuropsychopharmacology* 33 (2008): 513–23, doi/org.10.1038/sj.npp.1301443.

29. Herbert and Pollatos, "The Body in the Mind."

30. Ana Tajadura-Jimenez and Manos Tsakiris, "Balancing the 'Inner' and the 'Outer' Self," *Journal of Experimental Psychology: General* 143, no. 2 (2014): 736–44, doi.org/10.1037/a0033171.

Chapter 6. Building Body Awareness

1. Daniel Goleman and Richard Davison, *Altered Traits: Science Reveals How Meditation Changes Your Mind, Brain, and Body* (New York: Avery, 2017).

2. Susan Sands, "Less Time Ahead, More Behind," *Women and Therapy* 32 (2009): 158–69, doi.org/10.1080/02703140902851948.

3. Mind and Life Institute and the Awake Network Foundation, Science and Wisdom of Emotions Summit, May 2–5, 2021, scienceandwisdomofemotions.com.

4. Norman Farb et al., "Interoception, Contemplative Practice, and Health," *Frontiers in Psychology* 6, no. 763 (2015): 3–26, doi.org/10.3389/ffpsygg.2015.00763.

5. Farb et al., "Interoception, Contemplative Practice, and Health."

6. Farb, ibid.

7. Anil Seth, Keisuke Suzuki, and Hugo Critchley, "An Interoceptive Predictive Coding Model of Conscious Presence," *Frontiers in Psychology* 2 (2011): 395, doi.org/10.3389/fpsyg.2011.00395.

8. Cynthia Price, "Body-Oriented Therapy in Recovery from Child Sexual Abuse: An Efficacy Study," *Alternative Therapies in Health and Medicine* 11, no. 5 (2005): 46–57.

9. Matthieu Ricard, Antoine Lutz, and Richard Davidson, "The Mind of the Meditator," *Scientific American* 311, no. 5 (2014): 38–45.

10. Sharon Salzberg, *Lovingkindness: The Revolutionary Art of Happiness* (Boulder, CO: Shambala Classics, 2002).

11. Lewis Richmond, *Aging as a Spiritual Practice* (New York: Gotham, 2012).

12. Ricard et al., "The Mind of the Meditator."

13. Jon Kabat-Zinn, *Full Catastrophe Living*, rev. ed. (New York: Bantam, 2013).

14. Wolf Mehling, Cynthia Price, Jennifer Daubenmier, et al., "The Multidimensional Assessment of Interoceptive Awareness (MAIA)," *PLOS ONE* 7, no. 11 (2012): doi.org/10.1371/journal .pone.0048230.

15. Norman Farb, Zindel Segal, and Adam Anderson, "Mindfulness Meditation Training Alters Cortical Representations of Interoceptive Attention," *Social, Cognitive, and Affective Neuroscience* 8, no.1 (2013): 15–26, doi.org/10.1093/scan/nss066.

16. Sahib Khalsa et al., "The Practice of Meditation Is Not Associated with Improved Interoceptive Awareness of the Heartbeat," *Psychophysiology* 57, no. 2 (February 2020): e13479, doi.org/10.1111 /psyp.13479.

17. J. David Cresswell et al., "Brief Mindfulness Meditation Training Alters Psychological and Neuroendocrine Responses to Social Evaluative Stress," *Psychoneuroendocrinology* 44 (June 2014): 1–12, doi.org/10.1016/jpsyneuen.2014.02.007.

18. Thomas Gorman and C. Shawn Green, "Short-Term Mindfulness Intervention Reduces the Negative Attentional Effects Associated with Heavy Media Multitasking," *Scientific Reports* 6, no. 24542 (2016), doi.org/10.1038.srep24542.

19. Antoine Lutz et al., "Regulation of the Neural Circuitry of Emotion by Compassion Meditation," *PLOS One* 3, no. 33 (2008), doi.org/10.1371/journal.pone.0001897.

20. Mark Williams et al., "Mindfulness-Based Cognitive Therapy for Preventing Relapse in Recurrent Depression," *Journal of Consulting and Clinical Psychology* 82, no. 2 (2014): 275–286, doi.org/10 .1037/a0035036.

21. Goleman and Davidson, *Altered Traits*.

22. Robert Keith Wallace et al., "The Effects of the Transcendental Meditation and TM-Siddhi Program on the Aging Process," *International Journal of Neuroscience* 16, no. 1 (1982): 53–58, doi.org /10.3109/00207458209147602.

23. Eileen Luders, Nicholas Cherbuin, and Christian Gaser, "Estimating Brain Age Using High Resolution Pattern Recognition: Younger Brains in Long-Term Meditation Practitioners," *NeuroImage* 134 (July 1, 2016): 508–13, doi.org/10.1016/j.neuroimage .2016.04.007.

24. Sara Lazar et al., "Meditation Experience Is Associated with Increased Cortical Thickness," *Neuroreport* 16, no. 17 (2005), ncbi.nim.nih.gov.

25. Goleman and Davidson, *Altered Traits*.

26. Melissa Rosenkranz et al., "Reduced Stress and Inflammatory Responsiveness in Experienced Meditators Compared to a Matched Healthy Control Group," *Psychoneuroimmunology* 68 (2016): 117–25, doi.org/10.1016/jpsyneuen.2016.02.013.

27. Elizabeth Hoge et al., "Loving-Kindness Meditation Practice Associated with Longer Telomeres in Women," *Brain Behavior and Immunity* 32 (2013): 159–63, doi.org/10.1016/j.bbi.2013.04.005.

28. Elissa Epel et al., "Can Meditation Slow Rate of Cellular Aging? Cognitive Stress, Mindfulness, and Telomeres," *Annals of the New York Academy of Sciences* 1172, no. 1 (2009): 34–53, doi.org/10 .1111/j.1749-6632.2009.04414.x.

29. Anthony Zanesco et al., "Cognitive Aging and Long-Term Maintenance of Attentional Improvements Following Meditation Training," *Journal of Cognitive Enhancement* 2, no. 1 (September 2018): 259–75, doi.org/10.1007/s41465-018-0068-1.

30. J. E. Raymond, K. L. Shapiro, and K. M. Arnell, "Temporary Suppression of Visual Processing in an RSVP Task: An Attentional Blink?" *Journal of Experimental Psychology: Human Perception and Performance* 18, no. 3 (1992): 849–60, doi.org/10.1037/0096-1523.18.3.849.

31. H. A. Slagter et al., "Mental Training Affects Distribution of Limited Brain Resources," *PLOS Biology* 5, no. 6 (June 2007), doi.org/10.1371/journal.pbio.0050138.

32. Sara Van Leeuwen, Notger Mueller, and Lucia Melloni, "Age Effects on Attentional Blink Performance in Meditation," *Consciousness and Cognition* 18, no. 3 (September 2009): 593–99, doi.org/10.1016/jconcog.2009.05.001.

33. Lorenza Colzato et al., "Meditation-Induced States Predict Attentional Control over Time," *Consciousness and Cognition* 37 (December 2015): 57–62, doi.org/10.1016/j.concog.2015.08.006.

34. Gill Livingston et al., "Dementia Prevention, Intervention, and Care," *Lancet* 390, no. 10113 (2017): 2673–2734, doi.org/10.1016/S0140-6736(17)31363-6.

35. Chengxuan Qui and Laura Fratiglioni, "Aging Without Dementia Is Achievable: Current Evidence from Epidemiological Research," *Journal of Alzheimer's Disease* 62, no. 3 (2018): 933–42, doi.org/10.3233/JAD-171037.

36. Qui and Fratiglioni, "Aging Without Dementia Is Achievable."

37. Melanie Huttenrauch, Jose Lopez-Noguerola, and Susana Castro-Obregon, "Connecting Mind-Body Therapy-Mediated Effects to Pathological Features of Alzheimer's Disease," *Journal of Alzheimer's Disease* 82, s. 1: S65–S90, doi.org/10.3233/JAD-200743.

38. James Nestor, *Breath: The New Science of a Lost Art* (New York: Riverhead, 2020).

39. Alice Meuret et al., "Hypoventilation Therapy Alleviates Panic by Repeated Induction of Dyspnea," *Biological Psychiatry: Cognitive Neuroscience and Neuroimaging* 3, no. 6 (June 2018): 539–45, doi.org/10.1016/j.bpsc.2018.01.010.

40. Stephen Porges, *The Pocket Guide to the Polyvagal Theory* (New York: Norton Professional Books, 2017).

41. Herbert Benson, *The Relaxation Response* (New York: Random House, 1982).

42. Wim Hof, *The Wim Hof Method* (Boulder, CO: Sounds True, 2020).

43. Lois Baker, "Lung Function May Predict Long Life or Early Death," University of Buffalo News Center, September 12, 2000, buffalo.edu/news/releases/2000/09/4857.html.

44. William J. Broad, *The Science of Yoga: The Risks and the Rewards* (New York: Simon and Schuster, 2012).

45. Broad, *The Science of Yoga*.

46. Tiffany Field, "Yoga Clinical Research Review," *Complementary Therapies in Clinical Practice* 17, no. 1 (2011): 1–8, doi.org/1016/jctcp.2010.09.007.

47. Field, "Yoga Clinical Research Review."

48. Heather Houston, "The Art of Mindful Singing," heatherhoustonmusic.com.

49. Peter Wayne et al., "Effects of Tai Chi on Cognitive Performance in Older Adults," *Journal of the American Geriatric Society* 62, no. 1 (2014): 25–39, doi.org/10.1111/jgs.12611.

50. Jingling Yang et al., "Tai Chi Is Effective in Delaying Cognitive Decline in Older Adults with Mild Cognitive Impairment," *Evidence-Based Complementary and Alternative Medicine*, March 25, 2020, doi.org/101155/2020/3620534.

51. Fuzhong Li, John Fisher, and Peter Harmer, "Improving Physical Function and Blood Pressure in Older Adults Through Cobblestone Mat Walking," *Journal of the American Geriatrics Society* 53, no. 8 (August 2005): 1305–12, doi.org/10.1111/j.1532-5415.2005.53407.x.

52. Chris Crowley and Henry Lodge, *Younger Next Year for Women* (New York: Workman, 2004).

53. Ulf Ekelund et al., "Joint Associations of Accelerometer Measured Physical Activity and Sedentary Time with All-Cause Mortality: A Harmonized Meta-analysis in More Than 44,000 Middle-Aged and Older Individuals," *British Journal of Sports Medicine* 54, no. 24 (2020), doi.org/10.1136/bjsports-2020-103270.

54. Qing Li, *Forest Bathing: How Trees Can Help You Find Health and Happiness* (New York: Penguin, 2018).

55. Daniel J. Levitin, *Successful Aging: A Neuroscientist Explores the Power and Potential of Our Lives* (New York: Dutton, 2020).

56. Melanie Thernstrom, "My Pain, My Brain," *New York Times Magazine,* May 14, 2006.

57. Michael Pollan, *In Defense of Food: An Eater's Manifesto* (New York: Penguin, 2008).

58. Emeran Mayer, *The Mind-Gut Connection* (New York: Harper Wave, 2016).

59. Matthew Walker, *Why We Sleep: Unlocking the Power of Sleep and Dreams* (New York: Scribner, 2017).

60. Andrew Lim et al., "Sleep Fragmentation and the Risk of Incident Alzheimer's Disease and Cognitive Decline in Older Persons," *Sleep* 36, no. 7 (2013): 1027–32, doi.org/10.5665/sleep.2802.

61. Shahrad Taheri et al., "Short Sleep Duration Is Associated with Reduced Leptin, Elevated Ghrelin, and Increased Body Mass Index," *PLOS Medicine* 1, no. 3 (2004), doi.org/10.1371/journal .pmed.0010062.

62. Eric Stice et al., "Weight Gain Is Associated with Reduced Striatal Response to Palatable Food," *Journal of Neuroscience* 30, no. 39 (2010): 13105–09, doi.org/10.1523/JNEUROSCI.2105-10.2010.

Chapter 7. Our Aging Bodies, Our Aging Selves

1. Daniel J. Levitin, *Successful Aging: A Neuroscientist Explores the Power and Potential of Our Lives* (New York: Dutton, 2020).

2. Gene Cohen, *The Creative Age: Awakening Human Potential in the Second Half of Life* (New York: Avon, 2000).

3. Sunghan Kim, Lynn Hasher, and Rose Zacks, "Aging and a Benefit of Distractibility," *Psychological Bulletin* 14, no. 2 (2007): 301–05, doi.org/10.3758/bf03194068.

4. Laura Carstensen, *A Long Bright Future* (New York: Public Affairs, 2009).

5. Jonathan Rauch, *The Happiness Curve* (New York: Picador, 2019).

6. Michael Thomas et al., "Paradoxical Trend for Improvement in Mental Health with Aging: A Community-Based Study of 1,546 Adults Aged 21–100 Years," *Journal of Clinical Psychiatry* 77, no. 8 (August 2016): 1019–25, doi.org/10.4088/JCP.16m10671.

7. Levitin, *Successful Aging*.

8. Susan Sands, "Less Time Ahead, More Behind," *Women and Therapy* 32 (2009): 158–69, doi.org/10.1080/02703140902851948.

9. Erik Erikson, *Childhood and Society* (New York: W. W. Norton, 1950).

10. Heinz Kohut, "Forms and Transformations of Narcissism," *Journal of the American Psychoanalytic Association* 14 (1966): 243–72, doi.org/10.1177/000306516601400201.

11. Carstensen, *A Long Bright Future*.

12. Sands, "Less Time Ahead."

13. Danielle Quinodoz, *Growing Old: A Journey of Self-Discovery* (New York: Routledge, 2010).

14. Erikson, *Childhood and Society*, 268.

15. Quinodoz, *Growing Old*, 6.

16. Anaïs Nin, from her diary; see Carol A. Dingle, ed., *Memorable Quotations: French Writers of the Past* (Lincoln, NE: Writers' Club Press, 2000).

17. Igor Grossmann et al., "Reasoning About Social Conflicts Improves into Old Age," *Proceedings of the National Academy of Sciences USA* 107, no. 16 (2010): 7246–50, doi.org/10.1073/pnas.1001715107.

18. Laura Carstensen et al., "Emotional Experience Improves with Age: Evidence Based on over 10 Years of Experience Sampling," *Psychological Aging* 26, no. 1 (2011): 21–33.

19. Sands, "Less Time Ahead."

20. Elliott Jacques, "Death and the Mid-life Crisis." *International Journal of Psychoanalysis* 46, no. 4 (1965): 502–14.

21. Colarusso, "Developmental Time Sense."

22. Gisela Labouvie-Vief, "Dynamic Integration Theory: Emotion Cognition and Equilibrium in Later Life," in *Handbook of Theories of Aging*, ed. Vern Bengston et al. (New York: Springer, 2009), 277–93.

23. Harry Stack Sullivan, *Conceptions of Modern Psychiatry* (Washington, DC: William Alanson White Psychiatric Foundation, 1947), 7.

24. Marian Diamond, David Krech, and Mark Rosenzweig, "The Effects of an Enriched Environment on the Histology of the Rat Cerebral Cortex," *Journal of Comparative Neurology* 123, no. 4 (1964), doi.org/10.1002/cne.901230110.

25. Cohen, *The Creative Age*.

26. Cohen, ibid.

27. Cohen, 13.

28. B. L. Miller et al., "Emergence of Artistic Talent in Frontotemporal Dementia," *Neurology* 51, no. 4 (1998): 978–82, doi.org/10.1212/WNL.51.4.978.

29. George Vaillant, *Aging Well: Surprising Guideposts to a Happier Life* (New York: Little, Brown, 2002).

30. Ed Diener and Martin Seligman, "Very Happy People," *Psychological Science* 13, no. 1 (2002), doi.org/10.1111/1467-9280.00415.

31. Vaillant, *Aging Well.*

32. Chengxuan Qui and Laura Fratiglioni, "Aging Without Dementia Is Achievable: Current Evidence from Epidemiological Research," *Journal of Alzheimer's Disease* 62, no. 3 (2018): 933–42, doi.org /10.3233/JAD-171037.

33. J. Holt-Lunstad et al., "Loneliness and Social Isolation as Risk Factors for Mortality: A Meta-Analytic Review," *Perspectives on Psychological Science* 10, no. 2 (2015): 227–37; *Washington Post,* October 4, 2017.

34. Barbara Kingsolver, *Animal Dreams* (New York: HarperCollins, 1990).

35. N. Maestas, "Back to Work: Expectations and Realizations of Work after Retirement," *Journal of Human Resources* 45, no. 3 (2010): 718–48.

36. Valory Mitchell, "Who Am I Now? Using Life Span Theories in Psychotherapy in Late Adulthood," *Women and Therapy* 32, nos. 2–3 (2009): 298–312, doi.org/10.1080/02703140902851930.

37. Carstensen, *A Long Bright Future.*

38. Laurie Santos, "The Science of Well-Being" (online course), Yale University, coursera.org.

39. Sonja Lyubomirsky et al., "Becoming Happier Takes Both a Will and a Proper Way," *Emotion* 11, no. 2 (2011): 391–402, doi.org /10.1037/1150952.

40. Elizabeth Dunn, Laura Aknin, and Michael Norton, "Spending Money on Others Promotes Happiness," *Science* 319, no. 5870 (2008): 1687–88, doi.org/10.1126/science.1150952.

41. Margaret Cruikshank, *Learning to Be Old: Gender, Culture, and Aging* (Lanham, MD: Rowman & Littlefield, 2009), 2.

42. J. L. Burke, "Young Children's Attitudes and Perceptions of Older Adults," *International Journal of Aging and Human Development* 14, no. 3 (1981–1982): 205–22, doi.org/10.2190/4j7n-rg79-hjqr-fldn.

43. Becca Levy et al., "Longevity Increased by Positive Self-Perceptions of Aging," *Journal of Personality and Social Psychology* 83, no. 2 (2002): 261–70, doi.org//10.1037//00.

44. Becca Levy et al., "A Culture-Brain Link: Negative Age Stereotypes Predict Alzheimer's-Disease Biomarkers," *Psychological Aging* 31, no. 1 (2016): 82–88, doi.org/10.1037/pag0000062.

45. Becca Levy et al., "Association Between Positive Age Stereotypes and Recovery from Disability in Older Persons," *JAMA* 308, no. 19 (2012): 1972–73, doi.org/10.1001/jama.2012.14541.

46. Erdman Palmore, "The Ageism Survey: First Findings," *Gerontologist* 41, no. 5 (2001): 572–75, doi.org/10.1093/geront/41.5.572.

47. Levy et al., "Longevity Increased by Positive Self-Perceptions of Aging."

48. Boston Women's Health Collective, *Our Bodies, Ourselves* (New York: Simon and Schuster, 1973).

49. Ed Diener et al., "Subjective Well-Being: Three Decades of Progress," *Psychological Bulletin* 125 (March 1999): 276–302, doi.org/10.1037/0033-2909.125.2.276.

50. M. C. Carlson et al., "Impact of the Baltimore Experience Corps Trial on Cortical and Hippocampal Volumes," *Alzheimer's and Dementia* 11, no. 11 (2015): 1320–48, doi.org/10.1016/j.jalz.2014.12.005.

51. Gloria Steinem, Boston Speaker Series, Boston, MA, January 9, 2019, bso.org. Quoted in Levitin.

Index

Index

Acknowledgments

I could thank every woman I know whose body is aging or whose body I saw aging, starting with my stoic grandmother, Eugenie Wuichet, and my mother, Jean Sands. I've absorbed so much of what I know from so many bodies. Some of you, however, were particularly instrumental in bringing this book to life, and to you I offer my special gratitude:

My developmental consultant, Dorothy Wall, astutely helped me figure out what I wanted to say and how to craft it gracefully into a proposal. Felicia Eth, my tough and savvy literary agent, brilliantly helped me reconceive the book and stayed right with me all the way. Thanks also to literary agent Diana Finch for her assistance in refining an earlier proposal.

The people at Sounds True really *are* a lot kinder than most people. My inspiring editor, Jennifer Yvette Brown, has such a deft ear for language and deep understanding of women's issues. Production editor Laurel Szmyd effortlessly kept all plates spinning while offering abundant reassurance. Thanks also to all the talented designers, copyeditors, and squadrons of people it takes to produce a book.

Special thanks to my most generous friend Saul Rosenberg, who carefully read the entire manuscript at the very last minute and offered incisive and invaluable suggestions. Dorty Nowak suggested important changes in early chapters and dreamed up the title, *The Inside Story*, one night over dinner. Linda Blachman provided aging expertise and loving support from the very beginning. When my resolve was wavering, Frances Verrinder was always there to add steel to my backbone. Other people who generously offered interviews, invaluable ideas, or support include Patricia Hart, Terry Schulman, Shawnee Cuzillo, Claudia Toomey, Shan Guisinger, Marsha Hebden, Arlene Noble, Cindy Sachs, Laura Mason, Melissa Holub, Maureen Franey, Mei Mei Spalding, Nancy Davis, Adrianne Feldstein, Susan Fadley, Elizabeth Watson, Janet Berrien, and Diana Murray.

I also want to thank my psychoanalytic colleagues and mentors, particularly the late Philip Bromberg, Robert Stolorow, Peter Goldberg, and Jean Petrucelli, for their generative ideas on the body/mind, my superb neuroscience instructor Maggie Zelner, and the teachers at Spirit Rock Meditation Center.

I am deeply grateful to my patients, many of whom appear in disguised form in this book, who have courage to open up their hearts and minds to me.

Finally, I want to thank my husband, Fred, for his understanding and fine cooking during my years of writing preoccupation, and to my son, Dan, and daughter-in-law, Jessica, for providing joy throughout.

About the Author

S usan Sands, PhD, is an internationally recognized clinical psychologist, best known for her articles and presentations on eating disorders and body image, as well as on aging, trauma, female development, and mind-body integration. She has been called one of eight "trailblazers . . . in our understanding of eating disorders and bodies."[1] Dr. Sands is on the faculty of the Psychoanalytic Institute of Northern California (PINC) and is an assistant clinical professor at UC Berkeley. Earlier, she worked in the field of journalism as a reporter, writer, and editor, including posts at *Newsweek* and the *Saturday Review*. Her long-term interest in Buddhist thought and meditation has also been an important influence. Dr. Sands lives in Berkeley, California, where she maintains a private practice in psychotherapy and supervision of other therapists. She can be reached at susanhsands@gmail.com.

---

1   Introduction, *Body-States*, ed. Jean Petrucelli (New York: Routledge, 2015).

About Sounds True

Sounds True is a multimedia publisher whose mission is to inspire and support personal transformation and spiritual awakening. Founded in 1985 and located in Boulder, Colorado, we work with many of the leading spiritual teachers, thinkers, healers, and visionary artists of our time. We strive with every title to preserve the essential "living wisdom" of the author or artist. It is our goal to create products that not only provide information to a reader or listener but also embody the quality of a wisdom transmission.

For those seeking genuine transformation, Sounds True is your trusted partner. At SoundsTrue.com you will find a wealth of free resources to support your journey, including exclusive weekly audio interviews, free downloads, interactive learning tools, and other special savings on all our titles.

To learn more, please visit SoundsTrue.com/freegifts or call us toll-free at 800.333.9185.

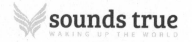

sounds true
WAKING UP THE WORLD